THE MAKING OF A VETERINARIAN

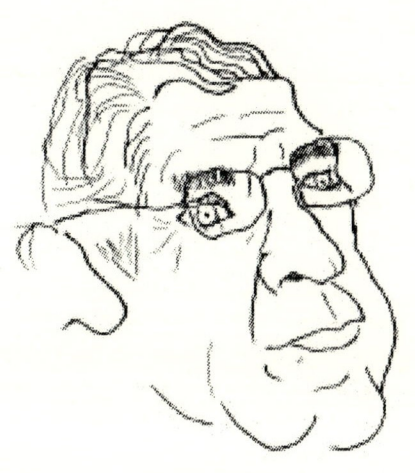

D.J. "Doc" McDermith

Copyright © 2002 by D.J. McDermith
All rights reserved.

No part of this manuscript may be reproduced or transmitted in any form or by any electronic or mechanical means, including photocopying, recording or by any information storage and retrieval system, without the written permission of the writer, D.J. McDermith, as provided by The Copyright Protection Law of The United States, Title 17, U.S. Code, Section 106 ofthe 1976 Copyright Act.

For information:
Open Book Publishing
Rt. 2 Box 2607
Birch Tree, MO 65438

First Open Book Edition 2002

ISBN 0-97191-671-3

Cover and book design by Lisa Fann

Printed in the United States of America

To my three sons Monte, Scott, and Roger

A RETIRED COUNTRY VETERINARIAN GOES TO WORK!

When Dr. McDermith moved to Summersville, Missouri from Illinois, he thought he was moving to the Ozarks to relax, raise cattle, and ride his horses. But, as soon as the people around Summersville found out he was a veterinarian, they put the "Retired Veterinarian to work"!

I have known Dr. McDermith for the last 20 years. We have practiced veterinary medicine in adjoining counties and over the years have become very good friends. Many times we have consulted with each other about problem cases.

Dr. McDermith has a pleasant personality and I have always enjoyed being around him to listen to his humorous stories and experiences during his practice. He was always a very ethical and professional veterinarian.

D.J. "Doc" McDermith

A heart attack forced Dr. McDermith to reduce his work load. People around Summersville began to realize how valuable he was to the community.

Janie, his late wife, was very helpful to him in his practice. If she wasn't helping him on a country call, she was answering the phones.

After reading this book I found it very interesting and humorous. As a practicing veterinarian, I can relate to his experiences and feel that everyone, young and old, will enjoy this book.

--Dr. Ireatess C. Keeney

The Making of a Veterinarian

INTRODUCTION

This is not a scientific book. This is a story of how a poor country boy became impressed with his local veterinarian and decided to pursue a veterinary degree even though livestock farming was his first love.

A good relationship has always been maintained with my clients and business friends. A drug salesman who called on us for nineteen years named Lee Kertlink from Hannibal, Missouri, would come every five weeks on Thursday at noon. He would go on calls with us until we finished that night. When he retired he told me that when I went to a farmer's place, whether the animal lived or died, the farmer was in a better mood when we left than when we got there. I think that was a compliment.

I met my boys, my grandkids, and my great grandkids at Ryan's restaurant in Effingham, Illinois, a while back for Sunday lunch. A young man came to our table and was visiting with my son Roger. I didn't recognize him but I was raised neighbors to his mother's family and did vet work for them for years. His name was Bruce Probst, a local veterinarian, and his brother Allen is also a veterinarian. Bruce said I was responsible for him going to vet school. He said I always seemed to be having fun so that's what he wanted to do.

Below is a letter from a friend that I think demonstrates the appreciation that people have shown me over the years.

```
                    Vandalia Ill
                    April 23 1967

D.J.McDermith
Kind Friend
                Enclosed You Will find A picture
You And your office girl ha ha
sorry I dident hold camera just a little
higher asialmost missed you Please excuse
my poor typing I ▬▬▶ Think You are a
Wonderfull veterinary and a nice ▬▬▬person
    I think of the times we called you day
or night and you come 30 mi  to our home
I meen  every woord Of it
i will send you apicture of a clane so if
the rats get to bad  you can scare them
      with it
            A Friend
                Blankenship,s & Klan,s
```

The Making of a Veterinarian

Many of my experiences have been interesting and funny, as I have tried to relate in this book.

I thank God I was able to make a decent living doing the things and dealing with the people I loved most. Farmers are truly the salt of the earth.

The Making of a Veterinarian

STRAUSS PLACE 1925-1928

I was born on August 29, 1927, about a mile North of Ohlman, Illinois to Jesse and Mabel McDermith. Dad always said I was born during wheat sowing time. He called me "Bub" unless he was mad, then he called me "Donald."

Kenneth Barringer lived at the Strauss place several years after we moved away. Ken was a good farmer and kept his farm neat.

Dad was a plain dirt farmer for several years. Most farm renters moved pretty often, I'm not sure why. I guess farmers were looking for a better farm and owners were looking for a better farmer. Some owners and farmers just couldn't get along.

Dad was from a family of fifteen children. His dad, Scott, was married to Elizabeth Petijohn. They had two boys (Guy and Orville). Elizabeth died, and Scott then married Etta Cozart. They had two boys and one girl (Loyal, Jim and Letha), before Scott lost his second wife. He then married Julia Hadley, Dad's mother. Julia had been married before, and was widowed with three girls (Annis, Verna, and Ethel). Scott and Julia had five boys and two girls (Virgil, Jesse, Emma, Clark, Kenneth, Harry, and Opal). Dad said they always had fried chicken on Sundays and special occasions. I'm sure Dad was joking but he said he was eighteen years old before he knew a chicken had anything but a neck.

My mother, Mabel Howerton, was from a family of four girls and one boy. The boy was hit and killed by a car when he was twelve years old. As you can see, I have been blessed with uncles and aunts.

Dad grew up around Cowden, Illinois. His dad, Scott, died a few years before I was born. He passed away with pneumonia, around corn shucking time. I think Dad helped his mother for a year or so, then married and started farming for himself on the Strauss place. Everyone moved in March. All the crops were harvested and it was almost time to start sowing oats, etc. We moved to Pence place east of Pana in the spring after I was born.

The Making of a Veterinarian

PENCE PLACE 1928-1932

The Pence Place was east of Pana about a mile, then north, up a lane. The farm was poor ground with lots of gullies which tore up lots of machinery.

My sister Phyllis Carline was born May 27, 1929. Mom and I went to Jacksonville, where her folks lived, to have Sis. A week or two after she was born, Dad came up to bring them home. I was playing in the back yard and Dad came to see me before he went in to see Mom and my baby sis. I don't think he ever did live that down.

My folks met lots of fine people around Pana and they remained friends with them for years to come. Joe Warren was one of Dad's best friends. Dad said that if you picked Joe up as he was walking to town, by the time you got there Joe would convince you he was doing you a favor!

One Monday morning, when I was just past one year old, my mother was doing the wash and I was playing in the yard. I got out of the yard and into the corn field. I came out on the highway, a quarter mile from the house. Four businessmen in a Model T picked me up and took me to the house. By that time my mother had missed me. She had searched in the horse tank, the well and every place else she thought I might be. She told me later that, when we got there, she grabbed me from the men and ran in the house without ever thanking them.

Another friend of Dad's was Speedy Pfau who lived in Pana. He sold the restaurant he had run for years. One day he was standing on a corner waiting to cross when Dad stopped and asked him if he wanted to take a ride. The next week the story was in the paper.

Warning to Those Well Dressed and Not Busy

Ennis "Speedy" Pfau, longtime Pana character who once worked for a living ("Speedy's" eatin' joint which evaporated when it lost its ancient and established location) and now, he reports, and apparently, subsides on the percentage of the deals in certain more or less suspect real estate transactions, moped about the prominent places downtown last week, as is his wont, doing little in a nice, clean outfit of clothes unsullied by the sweat of honest toil. He looked pretty good.

Along drove equally nicely accoutred Jesse McDermith, well-to-do retired farmer and stock raiser, who noting the idle "Speedy" slowed to a typical Pfau speed (0 miles per hour) and said "Jump In."

"Speedy" got in, with less alacrity than his nickname indicates.

Along about the lake east of town, too far for a guy like "Speedy" to recover afoot, Mr. Pfau asked Mr. McDermith, "Where we going?"

And Jesse replied, "To a funeral in Cowden."

So they went to the funeral in Cowden, and "Speedy" says that although he didn't know anybody there, the preacher spoke well of the deceased, and the music was nice.

BARRETT PLACE 1930-1932

The Barrett place was about four miles North of Ohlman and one mile North of the Bear Creek road. At that time in our lives, we had no money. There wasn't any money. We had a house, a barn, a hen house and an old narrow garage. One memory I carry with me about the place is looking through the yard fence and crying every time Dad went to the barn or field.

Ed Eiders, a neighbor of ours, lived in the next house west of us. Ed and Dad were great friends to the end. Dad used to tell the story about the time Ed's house was on fire. Dad rushed over to help, but the house was already past saving. Dad asked Ed if there was anything he could do. Ed said, "No, I just hate to see it go." Ed always said just what he thought.

D.J. "Doc" McDermith

WALTERS PLACE 1932-1935

Frank Johnson and Bob Folkerts had just inherited the Walters place when we moved there and they were nice landlords.

While living on the Walters Place, my brother James William McDermith was born January 24, 1933.

Times were still hard. I remember Dad letting our 15-30 International tractor go back to the implement dealer. The banker and someone connected with the bank came by, and after reviewing everything, they advised Dad to take bankruptcy. They appreciated how he had tried but said it wasn't fair to his family to be strapped with this debt ($4000) that he couldn't pay. Dad never slept all night and the next morning he went into town and told them he would keep trying to pay it, and he did.

We had a half mile lane that was just dirt and would really get muddy in the winter. When we went some place dad would hitch "Old Worthy" to the car, then unhitch him at the end of the lane, tying him to the fencerow until we came home. Sometimes we would try it without a horse. When we couldn't go forward dad would back up and hit it again. One day my brother Jim, who was two years old, was riding with Dad on a sulky plow when Dad stopped to rest the horses. Jim looked up at my dad and said "Stuck? Back up!"

I started school at Sassafras school, which was about two miles west of where we lived. I learned to play several games at Sassafras, including "handy over" and "fox and the goose," which is played in the snow. Miss Lucille Miller was my first grade teacher and Logan Fern taught my second and third grade years.

At Christmas, during my first year of school, Dad got me an old pony, probably twenty-years-old, to ride to school. The first morning the neighbor lady came rushing out to see my pony and opened the gate for me to get out of the pasture onto the road. The second morning she happened to be in the yard and opened the gate again. The third morning I sat there on my pony and hollered for Mrs. Hunt. She finally came to the door and informed me that she wouldn't be opening the gate every morning! This was a good lesson for me.

One winter evening I was coming home on my pony. I had to ride around the garden to get to the barn and I was in a lope as usual. Dad told me then that my pony would slip and fall with me if I didn't slow down coming around the garden. A few evenings later I forgot to slow down. The ice had thawed on top, making it slippery, and down we went right on my foot. We were both mud from head to toe, and I always remembered to slow down after that.

Sis liked to sing and do recitals, and she furnished us with lots of entertainment around animals, mostly at her expense. One day my dad brought home a baby goat and, as goats can be, it was always into everything. One Sunday morning Sis was dressed to go to church and was on the front porch singing as usual, waiting for the rest of us to get ready. The goat slipped up behind her and when she saw it she fell off the porch. Her dress came down over the goats horns and there she was, dangling, because her feet couldn't touch the ground. The goat had all four feet braced with no intention of being pulled off the porch. It took the whole family to get Sis loose.

When any of us would cry Dad would call us a bawl-calf. One day when Sis was about four years old she asked to ride on the cultivator, which dad would often let us do, but he didn't trust the team and told her "no." Sis walked off sniffing and right quick she turned around and called Dad a bawl-calf, then went on to the house. Dad really got a laugh out of that.

My Dad liked fox terrier dogs and one day he got us kids a pup and we all thought the world of it. One morning Dad went to the barn to chore and when he opened the feedway door the pup shot by him and attacked a bucket calf. Dad scolded her and she quit, but she still acted kind of wild. A little later, while Dad was milking, he heard pigs squealing in the lot. It was the pup again. At that point, Dad caught her and locked her in the corncrib. The pup didn't act right the next morning so Dad decided to take her to the vet. Dad and Mom were in the front seat and Sis, Jim, the pup and I were all in the back seat. We took her to Dr. Singer in Pana, Illinois. He told my Dad right away to put her in the cage...she had rabies. Sure enough, he was right. The calf and several pigs died with it. Luckily she hadn't bit us kids.

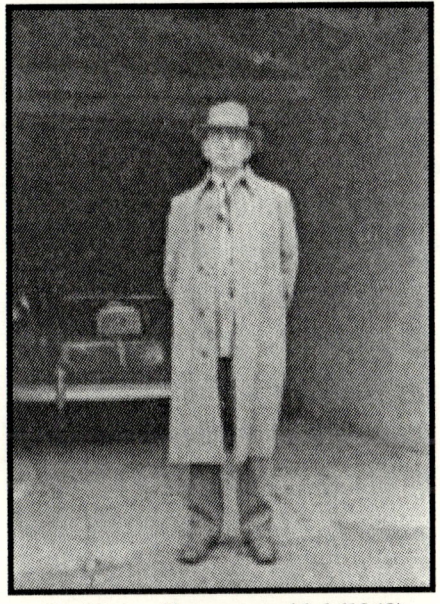

Dr. Henry Singer - my idol (1948)

In the fall of 1934 Dad realized several of the neighbors were in need of workhorses. They had gone to tractors but still needed horses to haul manure, to cultivate, and for other light jobs. They had stopped breeding their own, thinking the tractor would eliminate the need for horses. Dad went to the banker, Mr. Shriber, in Ohlman to borrow two or three thousand dollars to buy horses in the Dakotas. While Dad was waiting to see Mr. Shriber, Henry Klindworth, a well to do farmer in the area, was already in the office trying to borrow $800 to build a garage. Mr. Shriber turned him down. The walls were thin and Dad had heard their whole conversation. He considered just leaving but he didn't. When Dad presented his idea, Mr. Shriber was all for it and loaned him the money. Dad asked him why he had turned Henry down for $800, but let him (my dad) have two or three thousand that was very risky. After all, he knew Henry was a good man. Mr. Shriber said Henry didn't need that garage and he had to save that money for people that had to have it.

Dad did well with the horses, lots of them got sick, some had to be broke, but in the end, they made money. The next year Dad, Paul Turner and Joe Warren went to the Dakotas again. They bought two or three train carloads and sold them at auction in Springfield, Illinois. They made money then, too.

The Making of a Veterinarian

WARDELL PLACE 1936-1939

In 1936 we moved to the Wardell Place on Bear Creek Road. Dad was beginning to trade livestock and was gone from home more. He and Lloyd Barnes took Dad's tractor and Lloyd's threshing machine and did custom threshing in the neighborhood. Money was still in short supply. The two of them took baby calves, sorghum, and about anything else in payment for what they were owed. This led to a partnership that lasted seventeen years. Lloyd and Pauline raised Roger, their nephew, because he liked the farm life. We grew up together and had many memorable experiences.

Mr. Shroeder was tiling the Wardell farm and when they delivered the tile they laid the tiles along the fencerow. I was pulling Rog in a wagon, with my pony about that time. Mr. Shroeder saw us and said he would give us a quarter if we would haul the tile over to where he was digging in the field. Everything went fine until we started to divide the quarter. I thought I should have thirteen cents and Rog twelve cents because it was my pony and wagon. Rog agreed so I gave him twelve cents out of my bank, but he couldn't understand why I got the whole quarter. I tried to explain, but he got mad and walked the three miles home.

Sis and I went to Grant school, which was only about a quarter mile west on Bear Creek Road. Mildred McDowell was our teacher. She walked to school three miles and was a good strict teacher.

Charlie and Bertha Evans lived about a quarter mile East of us on Bear Creek Road. Charlie and Dad were raised neighbors down around Cowden. One day we were going to rake hay and the rake was gone. Dad remembered loaning it to Charlie the year before, so we went to check with him. He said, "Yes, I have it."

Dad asked, "Why didn't you bring it home?"

Charlie said he thought it was enough trouble for him to have had to come and get it.

Charlie's boy Francis was one year older than me and was my best friend. I had a small black Shetland pony and he had a little larger black Shetland pony. We were together most everyday.

We had some fine neighbors west on Bear Creek Road, Mr. and Mrs. Charlie Hitchcock. They had a Dodge Coupe car, which Mrs. Hitchcock usually drove. She was very short and could hardly see out, so she held her head high and let nothing distract her.

One morning I was on the right side of the oil road going to visit Francis. Francis was coming down the left side to see me. We both rode as fast as the ponies could gallop. I decided I would drive like Mrs. Hitchcock and not stop when we met. Francis had the same intentions. We were both riding bareback and, because the ponies were used to being together, when we met they both stopped in their tracks. We both went off over our ponies' heads. It took us a few days, but we finally healed up.

I loved my black pony "Major." His pitiful bridle had a rusty bent bit, with rotten leather that had been repaired in several places. To my delight, for Christmas one year I got a new pony bridle. I think that was my happiest Christmas. I kept Major in the hen house and when Dad and I went to do the chores I wanted to run over and show Major his new bridle. Dad sure got a kick out of that.

One day Dad came home with a beautiful four-year-old blue roan mare. She was just green broke with a very gentle nature. I had ridden her a couple of times and she was doing good. I asked Dad if she was broke double. He didn't know, so he set Sis up behind me, against her will. The mare got excited and wanted to buck, but I kept her from getting her head down. All at once she reared straight up. I hung on to the mane and Sis hung on to me and, luckily, she didn't fall over backwards. Dad didn't waste any time getting Sis off. With lots of riding the horse became a good, useful, reliable mare.

A short time later the mare got sick. We called Dr. Singer and he treated her for sleeping sickness. She got progressively worse over several days. We finally had to sling her. She recovered slowly. Dr. Singer said she would probably have brain damage and would be a "dummy" but she recovered completely and made a fine using mare. This was about the time I started developing respect for Dr. Singer.

While we lived on the Wardell place, the highway department made a farm to market blacktop road out of Bear Creek Road. It ran from Pana to the Nokomis-Taylorville black top.

They were building a bridge between our house and Grant school across a big drainage ditch and had blocked the main channel so they could work on the bridge and dig an eight foot channel across the road. I had a good gray stock horse named Polk-a-dot, and I had been checking the cattle every day for new calves, scours, pneumonia, etc. It came a big rain; water was everywhere. I couldn't get to the cows because they were on the other side of the drainage ditch, so I decided to swim Polk-a-dot across the drainage ditch before it crossed the narrow temporary channel. The current sucked us into the channel and I could see we were heading for a bunch of roots where the ditch turned on the other side of the road. I jumped and caught my elbows on the old roadbed and pulled myself out, but Polk-a-dot was still struggling in the roots. I thought he was sure going to drown. He finally got loose and came out on the road where I was. I was ashamed to have gotten him into that mess, but it never seemed to bother him.

John Morrison had worked for Dad for several years. He was a good fellow but pretty old and pretty cranky. We had a young team of mules. I was going to water them and John told me not to...they might hurt me. I already had them untied when he jerked them away from me and I hit my elbow on the doorframe. That really upset me. When Dad came home that evening I told him if he would get rid of John I would build the fires and do the chores. He said "You're only eleven years old, you can't do that," but he found John a place to work and he was gone in three or four days. I had bit off a pretty big chew but I did it and Dad was proud of me.

Our family had a good standard-bred team. The first fieldwork I can remember doing was rolling corn with a corrugated roller when the corn was about two or three inches tall. Dad was always gone trading livestock and one day I had finished rolling the corn and was looking for something else to do.

Dad had plowed up our old hog lot and the ground was hard and there were clods and chunks of dirt up to a foot across. I decided that it should be rolled. The roller wasn't doing much good and it was so rough I could hardly stay on the roller. All at once we hit a big chunk. My right foot slipped off the frame and went between the roller and frame. It startled the horses and I was overbalanced to where I couldn't pull on the reins much. Thankfully, they didn't run off and I finally got my leg out. It was bruised and skinned up but not broken. After that I decided I would stick to rolling corn.

Dad was doing lots of horse-trading and some of the transactions were pretty amusing. Once, Dad drove up to a man's house that had a team to sell. The lady of the house told him her husband was at the barn. The man said he wanted $250 for the team, which had new leather halters. Dad offered $230 if he got the halters with the horses. The man invited Dad to the house for a cup of coffee and to check with his wife about the price. It was no trouble to tell she was the boss. They decided to sell, but without the new halters. The next morning Dad went to pick up the horses, but the lady said her husband wasn't going to sell them to him.

Dad said "That's okay, I don't know what made me think I could ever get that kind of money for them."

She followed Dad to the barn and told her husband to let Dad have those horses, and the new halters, too.

The Making of a Veterinarian

AUGUST SINGER PLACE
1939-1940

The August Singer Place, which belonged to Dr. Henry Singer's brother, was the first place that Dad bought. I was in heaven there. It was more rolling land and there was even some timber left around.

Jim, Sis, and I walked one mile west through the timber to Cardsgrove school. Mrs. Gladys Bottomely was our teacher and she was great.

Dad made lots of improvements on the place; built fences and developed a spring that watered the horses, cattle, and hogs.

I had a horse named Old Jim. He was a racking horse and a jumper. Old Jim could outrun every horse around except Roy Adkins' Old Babe. They took turns winning.

When we first got him I would ride him down the lane, turn and jump a four barbed wire fence into the pasture, and bring the milk cows up to the barn... until my Dad saw me do that. I hadn't even thought about what it might do to Old Jim if he didn't make it.

    I stayed all night with Dave Kessen, a neighbor boy, one night. The next morning we got on two of their ponies and went to get the milk cows. It was freezing and the ponies were full of life. Dave's pony ran under a long limb, Dave grabbed it and pulled it about ten feet and let it go. We were in a dead run and by the time I saw what was happening it was too late to do anything to avoid the limb. My face was already burning. The tip of the limb hit me right in the face. I've never had anything before or since hurt that bad.

    An old friend of Dad's, Clint Miller, had struck oil on his farm near Beecher City. He wanted to buy a farm so Dad sold him ours and we bought the Miles place just across the road.

The Making of a Veterinarian

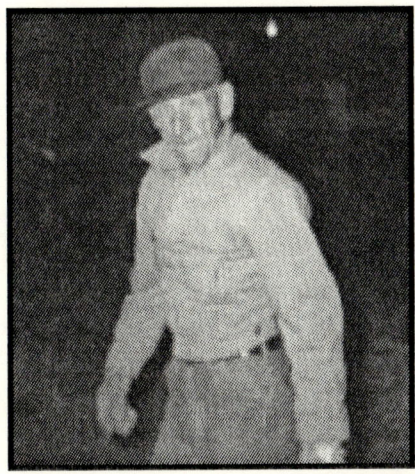

PeeWee Frailey, feeding the cattle, is surprised by the camera click.

MILES PLACE 1940-1957

The Miles Place had a new small barn and a beautiful old two-story house, but the land was worn out. Dad and Pee Wee (Logan Frailey), Dad's hired hand and distant cousin, plowed some of the gullies shut or smoothed them up. Jim and I hauled cobs home after school from the Rosamond elevator to fill the ditches. Dad and Pee Wee built seven ponds with a team and slip scraper to water the cattle and slow the water down.

We had a well broke team called Rex and Charlie. Our neighbor Dr. Roe, a retired dentist, was heavy on the booze. One evening he ran in the ditch at the end of our lane. Dad and PeeWee took the pickup out in the pasture to get Rex and Charlie to pull Doc out. PeeWee said he would just ride Charlie, and Rex would follow; no bridle, halter, or anything. Dad, always ready to play a trick on PeeWee, let them get started then took in after them in the truck. Peewee said his knees shook 'til he could hardly stand up when he got to the barn.

Some time later a neighbor from when we lived on the Walters place, Glenn Ryan, wanted to buy Rex and Charlie at a good price. PeeWee told Dad if they left he was leaving too. Dad sold them and, sure enough, PeeWee went and shucked corn for Glen for about a month and then he came back.

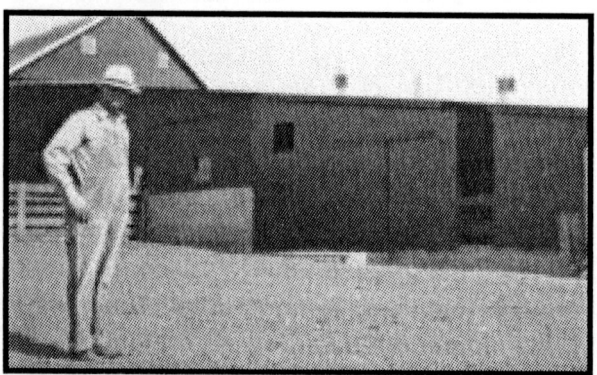

Jesse McDermith planning where to put a concrete silo, after adding on to the barn.

Lots of farmers depended on Dad to find them livestock and also to buy when they wanted to sell. Dad wanted to go to the Kansas City Stock Yards and buy a train carload of cows.

The Ohlman bank had closed and he would have to get the money from the Pana bank. He wasn't sure he could borrow that much so he talked to an old friend he had borrowed from before and he agreed to let him have it if the bank turned him down. Dad explained to the banker that he needed one carload and he thought they would cost between six and eight dollars per one hundred pounds. The banker told him to go ahead.

Dad stood around the yards all day and hadn't found anything that suited him. About the time Dad gave up and was starting to leave he noticed a bunch of cows being driven across an overhead alleyway. The man that owned them was following. Dad bought them for four dollars a hundred pounds. They had just had the calves weaned off them. They were thin and young, just what he wanted, but there were two carloads.

Dad was happy with his deal. The next morning he rushed in to tell the banker. The banker was mad because Dad bought two carloads instead of one.

That banker said "I'll just stop you before you get started, you'll spend a million dollars."

Dad said he would have the money by noon and would the banker please tell the seller as much if the seller called?

The banker said, "No, that would guarantee the money," and he wasn't going to do that. He wanted to know where Dad was getting the money.

As Dad started out the doors he said, "That isn't any of your business if you aren't going to loan the money to me. You're supposed to be so shrewd, you agreed to loan me the money to buy one carload at six to eight dollars per hundred pounds. I did a good job and bought two car loads for four dollars a hundred pounds which would be the same amount of money as one carload at eight dollars a hundred."

The banker said, "Jesse I'm not used to being talked to like that, but it does make sense. I'll loan you the money."

George Miller and his brother at Raymond, Illinois, were mule buyers. Dad had four mules he had bought down around Beecher City. One of them had a wart on his eyelid about the size of a walnut. It was so big that it almost pulled his eyelid shut. George said he would buy the three but he didn't want the one with the wart. Dad said that was a buck-brush wart and as soon as he was out of the buck-brush a while it would go away. Dad was kidding him but he believed it.

Dad saw him a couple of weeks later and he figured he would have to give him some money back on the mule. George asked Dad whether he had any trouble with that mule with the wart jumping out of the pasture. Dad said he hadn't.

George said, "Well, he's getting out and getting in the buck-brush somewhere because the wart is getting bigger every day."

Another time, Dad went to look at a group of weaned pigs a farmer had for sale. He had the pigs in a washhouse, which was built onto the back of the house. Dad said it didn't look like that would be healthy having the pigs so close to the house. The farmer said he didn't know he thought they had done about as good as any pigs he ever raised.

I started to high school in the fall of 1941. I had a '33 Chevy and hauled five neighbor kids to school. That's also about the time I started noticing girls.

I managed a date with a pretty redhead and Dad let me use his '41 Chevy. I was driving home about midnight and had to cross the railroad and go down highway 16 about a quarter mile then turn south down the brick pavement to go home. There was one car on route 16 about a half mile west, so I didn't stop at the stop sign. About a mile down the brick pavement a trooper named Slim Ethridge pulled me over and wanted to see my license. I told him I was only fifteen and didn't have any yet. He asked if I saw that stop sign. I said, "Yes, but there was just one car coming about a half mile back west."

He said, "Yes, that was me. Now, you take this car home and leave it there until you get your license."

Later when I was going to Illinois College at Jacksonville I would hitchhike home and that same trooper would always pick me up and bring me on home.

Dr. Singer, our vet, wore dark horn-rimmed glasses and they would slide down on his nose. One day he came and doctored a cow for Dad. The doctor gave Dad the bill for eight dollars. Dad got out a twenty, so the doctor got twelve dollars change. Dad just put it with the twenty dollars, and stuck it back in his billfold. They were pretty busy visiting during all of this, but Dad thought Doc Singer didn't act just right.

Dad asked, "Did I give you that twenty dollars, Doc?"

Doc looked up with his glasses slipped down and said, "No Jesse, you kept it all."

They laughed about that for years.

Another time we had a cow that had gotten into the ground corn. She was down, bloated and toxic before we found her. Dr. Singer came. He let off the gas, and pumped a gallon of oil in her. He was mixing two different kinds of medicine to give every two or three hours, when Dad asked if he thought she would make it.

Doc said, "No, she'll die."

"Why are you giving me all that medicine if she's going to die?" Dad asked.

Doc said, "It's customary, Jesse."

About thirty minutes after he left the cow died.

I thought that strange at the time, but now I realize occasionally an animal will live, even though you didn't feel it would.

~ ~ ~

My brother Jim was five years younger than me. One evening I went to the barn to chore and when I went into the feedway I could hear Jim talking in the back of the barn. We had a shorthorn heifer that liked to be petted and Jim was sitting on her rubbing her neck. I picked up a five-gallon bucket and tossed it under her trying to give her a scare. She jumped out from under Jim and he fell on the bucket. I wasn't very proud of that although he wasn't hurt bad.

The Making of a Veterinarian

In the fall of 1943 when I registered for my third year of high school, Mrs. Boone was my counselor. I had taken an extra subject every year. She said if I could take one more I could graduate in three years, so I did. My first year in College was really hard but with the help of good teachers, I made it. Mrs. Boone knew I planned to go to vet-school and thought she was doing me a favor, but I have wished many times I could have had that last year of high school.

The folks finished raising all three of us kids on the Miles farm. We had made a nice productive grass farm out of it. In 1957 Dad sold it to the Clavin brothers and moved to Nokomis.

D.J. "Doc" McDermith

ILLINOIS COLLEGE 1944-1945

I started taking pre-vet courses at Illinois College in Jacksonville, Illinois, in the fall of 1944. I fired the furnace in Dr. Black's home for my room as well as waited tables and washed dishes at Mrs. Vickery's three story boarding house.

I did well for about a month then I got some poor test scores...I couldn't concentrate and I was depressed.

I called home one evening and Mom answered. I hated to talk to her because she wanted me to get an education so badly. I asked her if they would come and get me, that I couldn't stand it another day. She said they would, but Dad wasn't home yet. We discussed it some more and finally she said if I would stay another day I could call the next evening if I still wanted to come home. Before we were through talking I knew I wasn't going home. I guess I was homesick, because when I found out they would come and get me the tension was gone.

I used to spend some weekends with Dr. Bolte, a veterinarian in Jacksonville, Illinois, which was good experience. My mother's sister, Violet, who was deaf, lived there and was a big help to me.

I bought a nice bay colt from a black friend of mine that lived a couple blocks from Dr. Black, the MD who I roomed with. I gave a hundred-fifty for the colt and sold him for two seventy-five. I guess I have some of my Dad in me.

I hitchhiked home several weekends. Almost every time Slim Ethridge, the state cop that caught me running the stop sign, would pick me up and take me home.

I used my Dad as a bank. When I needed money he would loan it to me, and when I had any I wasn't using, I sent it to him. We both kept track and there was no interest involved. When I started college I had ten cows and calves. Dad gave me $1125 for them. That and what I made working almost got me through two years of college.

D.J. "Doc" McDermith

TEXAS A & M

Just before I started Texas A&M I was home for a short time. Dad bought an eight hundred acre farm just about a mile south of us, which included the cattle, sows, and machinery. He knew I liked the farm. He told me he didn't want to influence me either way but if I would rather farm he would keep the eight hundred acres.

I didn't sleep much that night, but I decided if I got an education it would be hard to take away from me so I went back to school. Dad sold the whole works in about thirty days and made a decent profit.

Texas A&M was on a speed up program — three semesters in twelve months. I barely finished at Illinois College in time to start at A&M. Dad traveled with me on the train. We had to get off at Hearne, which was twenty-two or three miles from College Station and we had to walk a couple blocks from the station to get a taxi to take us the rest of the way.

On the way, we walked by a watermelon stand. It was hot and we decided to get a piece of melon. We were surprised when the fellow picked one up, split it and set the two halves in front of us. We pretty well cleaned it up but we didn't want much supper.

I didn't know A&M required students to be in the Corps, which was like being in the Army. I also didn't know it was an all boys school.

Dad and Dr. Marsteller, dean of the vet school, hit it off and they kept busy, looking at and talking about horses. Dad was leaving at six in the evening, the second or third day after we got there. I was wearing my uniform and was in ranks for the first time. Sergeants were yelling at us. I wondered then if I shouldn't be leaving with Dad. Before the year was over, I wished several times that I had left with him.

We were supposed to know just about everything there was to know about the College. If an upperclassman asked us a question we couldn't answer we had to say, "Sir, not being informed to the highest degree of accuracy I hesitate to articulate for fear I may deviate from the true path of rectitude." In short that meant, "Sir, I'm a dumb fish, Sir, I do not know, Sir."

I don't think I was really homesick, but I was lonely. I had met Mr. Miller who had a ranch about a mile from town and he raised Angus cattle. One Saturday afternoon I walked to his place and he showed me his cattle and his ranch. I found the bones from one of his horses that had died a year or two before. There was a burlap sack full. I cleaned them up and used them to study osteology.

Mr. Miller really knew how to entertain a farm boy and I sure appreciated him. One day I was visiting him and noticed there was a yellow Packard convertible sitting in his drive. Mr. Miller said it belonged to Dr. Hooper, a dentist in town who was hunting quail on his ranch.

After Mr. Miller and I had visited a while a young man came walking up. He had hunting boots, khaki pants rolled up a couple rolls, a loud shirt, a little narrow brimmed hat turned up all the way around, and a filtered cigarette holder that was eight or ten inches long. I thought he really looked strange. Later, he became one of my very best Texas friends. I rented pasture from him, we fed cattle in partnership and I castrated his bull calves.

A few years after I graduated I went back on the train again to A&M to a vet meeting. I stopped to see

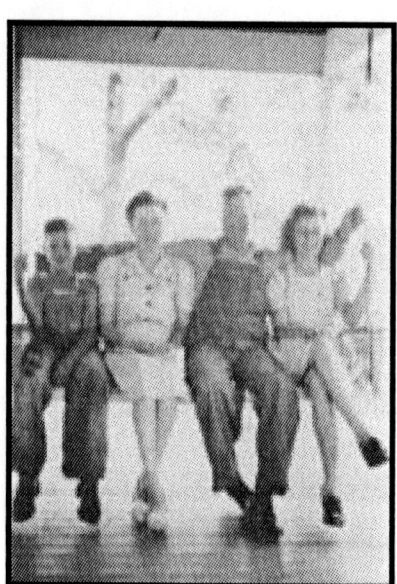

Jim, Mom, Dad & Phyllis on the front porch on the Miles Place. I was at Texas A&M.

The Making of a Veterinarian

Dr. Hooper for a minute. When I left he handed me the keys to his truck and told me to bring it by when I was leaving and Marge his wife would take me to the train. To me, that is a friend.

That year at A&M I didn't know from one day to the next if I would be called into military service. I had used up my $1125, and owed Dad $450. I decided to enlist so I could finish school on the GI Bill.

D.J. "Doc" McDermith

ARMY- INFANTRY- MEDICS
SEPTEMBER 1946 TO APRIL 1948

We went by train to Chicago and were sworn into the Infantry. Then we were sent to Camp Polk, Louisiana for sixteen weeks of basic training, which was very hard and humiliating. I guess it toughened me mentally and physically.

After basic we went to medical technician school in San Antonio, Texas. It was very interesting and helpful in my veterinary training later on.

After finishing med tech school several of us were sent to Germany. On the way over there I was a surgical technician on the ship.

Everything was pretty quiet until a 310 pound merchant marine with diabetes got appendicitis. They put off operating as long as they could, but finally throttled the ship down and headed into the wind to make it as smooth as possible.

The Making of a Veterinarian

He had evidently had an attack before because the appendix was adhered to the abdominal wall. While the doctors were trying to peal it loose, he stopped breathing. Four doctors did their best to save him but he didn't respond. I was behind his head holding his chin back to help his breathing. One of the doctors prepped and cut between my fingers to insert a tracheotomy tube, which was pretty exciting for my first surgical experience.

The next morning I helped do an autopsy, which was very interesting and exciting for me.

We landed in Bremmerhaven, then went to an infirmary at Schwabich Hall, which was about fifty miles from Stuttgart where we sent serious cases to the General hospital. Most of our work was minor injuries, venereal disease, and scabies. More severe injuries and diseases were sent to the hospital.

At that time penicillin was in beeswax. We had to heat it in the sterilizer then inject it in the buttocks with an inch and a half needle. Several would be waiting for their shot and every few days one of the patients would pass out and fall on the floor.

We had three medical technicians, two ambulance drivers, one doctor and one first sergeant. Each day we had sick call from seven to nine, then the ambulance went to Stuttgart.

One evening, two soldiers had turned a jeep over. We cleaned and bandaged them and I went with the ambulance. We were going down a mountain about sixty mph when all at once a rear tire started bumping. It took

D.J. "Doc" McDermith

about a half mile to get stopped and when we got out and looked, the inner tube was showing. Thank goodness it didn't blow.

Many days, when we finished sick call at nine a.m., we were through for the day. Sometimes I took the jeep to headquarters and sometimes I walked.

One day I took the jeep, got the mail, and went to the library until about eleven in the morning. At noon we all came out of the Infirmary heading for the mess hall, which was about a mile away. The jeep wasn't there and neither was Andy one of the ambulance drivers. We all gave Andy heck all the way to the mess hall and back.

That evening we came out to go to chow and the jeep still wasn't there. Everyone started cussing Andy and about that time he showed up. We were going to report it stolen if it wasn't there when we got back.

Then I remembered where the jeep was. I slowly dropped back and ran to headquarters, drove the jeep back to the Infirmary, and ran to the mess hall. No one knows, to this day, where it had been.

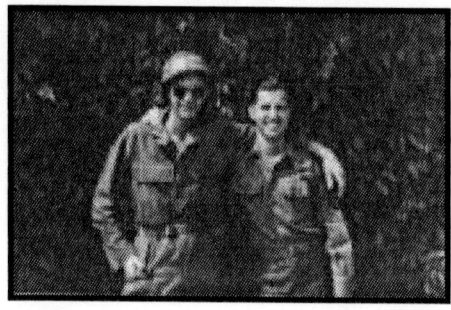

Bob Wock and Doc McDermith in Constabulary Medics in Germany. (1947)

The Making of a Veterinarian

Several of us were supposed to come home in March. A week or two before we were to leave we took an ambulance and went up in the mountains to ski. I fell the second trip and broke my leg, so I had to stay an extra month before I could come home.

It took eight days on the ship to come home and there was nothing to do but enjoy the ocean. We unloaded in New York.

I wanted to go to my uncles' house in Passaic, N.J. A cab driver wanted fifteen dollars to take me there, but I offered him five. He finally took me for six. I had a fine visit with Uncle Clark and his family, then took the train on to Illinois.

When I got home I had saved more money than the army had paid me. I didn't smoke so I sold my cigarettes (which cost $1.20) for twelve dollars at first, down to five dollars by the time I left. Also, we had a standard price to pull each other's duty. Every four nights we were on medical CQ or ambulance driver. They would pay $5 a night for medical CQ or $3 a night for ambulance driver. Several of the guys had German girlfriends they lived with and never pulled their night duty all the time we were there.

I had sent Dad $4800 and when I got home I bought a Frazer Manhattan for $4500. Dad said I was all front and no back, because I had a nice, expensive car and very little money.

In the fall of 1948, after Janey and I were mar-

D.J. "Doc" McDermith

ried, I traded the Frazier for a new Jeep to pull our house trailer to Texas so I could go to vet school again. Janey said I just kept the nice car until I got her to marry me then traded it for a Jeep.

MARRIED & WORKING WITH DR. SINGER

Janey and I had "gone together" since 1945. We courted mostly by letter and eventually married on June 25, 1948.

I came home from the Army in April of 1948 and couldn't get back in vet school until September. Janey worked at Ben Franklin in Pana and I worked for Dr. Singer.

I also broke eight horses to ride that summer. We would get up at three in the morning. I would ride one or two horses while she got dressed, fixed breakfast and packed our lunch. Then we would go just north of Pana to Smith's and ride another one, then go to work.

I enjoyed every day spent with Dr. Singer. He was a dedicated man, wonderful friend, and very amusing. He had a way of picking you up and carrying you all day long.

D.J. "Doc" McDermith

Dr. Singer bought eight-week-old, short-haired, mostly fox terrier pups for a pet shop in Chicago. He sent several crates every week. Their tails needed to be docked and healed.

One evening we came in late, after dark. A '35 Chevrolet Coupe was sitting in front of the office with a man and woman waiting in it. She was big and dressed in a very classy way with rouge and bright lipstick. He was a little dried up man with overalls and a straw hat. She told Doc they had some pups to sell. When he opened the trunk it was full of pups about twelve weeks old with big long tails. Doc said he couldn't use them. The lady tried three or four different approaches to get Doc to buy them but he simply had no place to go with them and turned them down.

When we got in the office and turned the light on Doc turned to me and said "Now that was a peculiar couple. She was a well-dressed lady and he was just a little hay-seed, but that was the way they presented themselves."

Doc Singer wore heavy horn-rimmed glasses and he had trouble keeping them up on his nose. He also smoked cigars until they were very short and chewed them for hours. Doc never drove himself anymore and he never complained about how I drove.

One day we were running late and I was driving about seventy-five on a black top road. The weeds were tall along side the road. About a hundred fifty feet ahead a shorthorn heifer jumped out in the road. There was no

The Making of a Veterinarian

telling which way she would go and I was trying my best to stop.

All at once she stuck her tail in the air and took down the road right in front of us. Her rear bobbed up and down in front of us for a long way then she turned back into the weeds.

We went about a mile and Doc raised his head to look at me over his sagging glasses. Laughing, he said, "She sure showed her ass!"

Coming in one evening about eight, we stopped in Tower Hill for gas at a filling station and grocery store. I was starved so I picked up a box of raisins. I opened them in the dark in the car on the way home. Doc and I ate about three quarters of the box. When we got in the office I poured out a handful and it was half worms. That almost made both of us sick. Needless to say, we didn't eat any more raisins for a while.

D.J. "Doc" McDermith

LAST THREE YEARS AT A&M
SEPTEMBER 1948 THRU JUNE 1951

My sophomore year was really hard, but that didn't keep me from doing other things while I should have been studying. Janey and I both worked in the veterinary pathology department for fifty cents an hour. My GI Bill paid around a hundred dollars a month.

I didn't have too good a record in parasitology. We had a big quiz coming up and I had really studied hard for it. I got along good on the quiz and went to the clinic where we were discussing the quiz. Every once in a while someone would mention something I didn't have on my test. All at once I knew something was wrong and I was in trouble.

I barely had time to get to the professor's office before five and, to my disappointment, he was gone when

I got there. Fortunately, I knew where he lived so I went to his house. Dr. Turk came to the door, and I nervously told him my problem.

I could tell he really didn't want to sort through those sixty-four papers but he did. He looked at the first page and the second page. Then he noticed that the third and fourth pages were stuck together and nothing was written on the fourth page. He gave me a choice to finish it or he would grade what I had with nothing off for what I skipped.

I told him we had been discussing the test and that I was so shook up I would rather he just grade what I had. He did, and I came out pretty good. I sure appreciated his fairness.

The first year back to college I traded horses. Some of them I trained and then hauled back to Illinois where Dad would sell them for me. We did good and the money helped pay some expenses. I should have been using that time to study, but it was hard to back away from things I had always loved.

One time I took a load of horses home over the weekend and brought a load of Holstein heifers back. I made some money, but got in trouble with the dean of vet school. I had forgotten we were supposed to register for the next semester that Saturday. I got a good talking to and had to stop some of my trading.

Every year Dr. Leonard hired two students (out of sixty-four) to work in the clinic. The third and fourth year Monte Swatzel and myself were hired, which to me was one of my greatest accomplishments. We were exposed to a wealth of experience through Dr. Leonard, and I enjoyed working with Monte and Dr. Leonard a great deal.

We worked every day, on weekends and on holidays, and it seemed like every day we learned something. I remember having two horses choke on watermelon rinds from different areas on the same day. I have never seen that before or since. Monte and I made seventy-five cents an hour, but we would have both worked for nothing.

One Saturday afternoon it came one of those gosling drownders. We had about everything treated and the clinic cleaned up. There were two wild Hereford cows in a little grass lot that needed retreating. I carried the medicine and Monte took the lariat. He caught one on the first throw but couldn't hold her on the wet grass. I had laid the medicine down to help him but it looked like he was water skiing, taking about twelve foot steps and jumping ditches. I laughed so hard that I couldn't help him, but he finally got her stopped.

When someone brought an animal to the clinic for treatment, either Monte, one of the clinic teachers, or I would get a history on the animal and the owner's name and address.

One day we were busy castrating horses and this old man came driving in past the office, the clinic, the cow barn and to the horse barn. He had brought a cow with gangrenous mastitis and had to have a teat cut off and some treatment for a few days. It wasn't until later that we realized the old man with his '36 Ford car and homemade trailer had driven off and none of us had gotten his name, address, or phone number.

Luckily, about the time the cow was ready to go home, he came driving back in. I helped him load the cow and told him to stop at the office, because we hadn't gotten his name, etc. He said he was G.R. Donahue, but that he would stop.

I rushed up to get the clipboard. He was crippled up and hard of hearing so I went out to the car. He told me again his name was G.R. Donahue. I told him I had that and asked his address and he said, "George."

I said, "Yes I have your name, but where do you live?"

He said, "George," so I showed him the clipboard where I had his name and showed him where I needed his address. He said, "Damn it, George." Come to find out, "George" was a little town about ten miles from the College. One store, three houses and a gas pump. I didn't tell everyone about that.

Our oldest son Monte was born January 11, 1951, before graduation in June of that year.

D.J. "Doc" McDermith

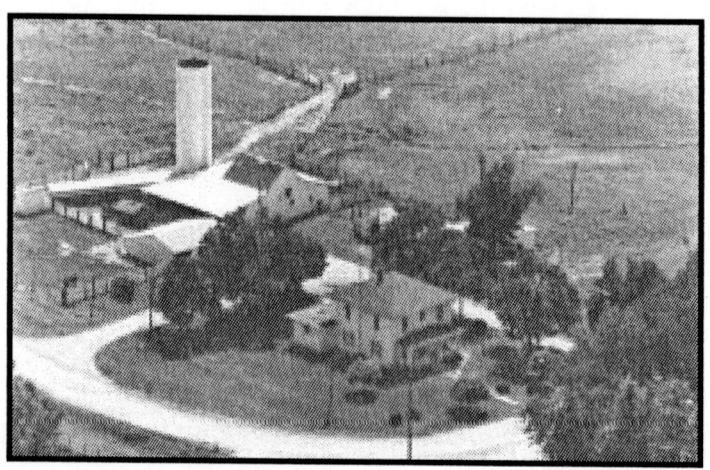

NOKOMIS: JOHN E. JOHNSON PLACE 1951-1970

When Janey and I moved from Texas back home to Illinois, we had our house trailer, a home made tandem stock trailer, 51 Ford car, 49 ford pickup, a Brahman bull and ten registered Angus heifers. I owed Dad $7000.

We bought a nice eleven-acre place in the east edge of Nokomis, for $16,000. It had a nice two-story house, two car garage, barn and henhouse. The house also had a nice basement which became my office for eight years. We had two small animal cages in the basement and seven more in a shed we fixed on the garage, with two outside runs alongside.

I had brought three registered American Saddle

Horses from Texas earlier. John E. Johnson, who I bought the place from, asked what I was going to do with them. I told him we planned to ride them, but if our business didn't take off we might have to eat them. He never forgot that. He always asked if I had eaten those horses yet.

Gordon Price, an auctioneer and cattle order buyer at Pana, Illinois, worked for me in the summer when he was in high school. One night about midnight a farmer called and had a cow trying to calve. She had already calved the day before and hid the calf in the pasture. She was now straining to pass the placenta so we went ahead and removed it. Fleas almost ate Gordon up on the way home. He is still complaining about that.

For eight years after getting out of school I castrated horses standing. I put on a demonstration at the University of Illinois veterinarian school. The horse bled worse than any I had ever done, which was embarrassing. The bleeding finally stopped without having to pack it. I finally went to anesthesia when a mule kicked the knife out of my hand and it flew about fifty feet.

It has been very interesting how farming has changed since 1951. Most farmers had 100 to 150 hens, 15 beef cows, six to fifteen milk cows, three or four sows and three or four horses. These farmers made good solid clients and were nice to work for.

I practiced five years alone, five years with Dr. Allen Port, then two years alone, two years with Dr. Jim Withers, then five more years alone. Also, I spent two years helping Dr. Lacey part time.

D.J. "Doc" McDermith

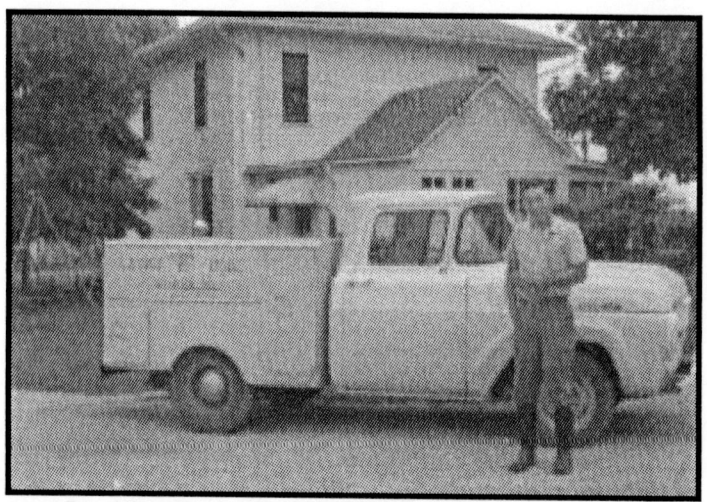

Dr. Allen Port was a Cornell graduate from New York.

My first year of practice I grossed $24,000. The fifth year I had increased it to $56,000. In five years Dr. Port and I increased the gross to $100,000. The next two years by myself it went to $120,000, which Dr. Withers and I maintained the next two years and I maintained the last five years.

Dr. Allen Port was a Cornell graduate and was from New York. Even though some of his New York ways were hard for midwest farmers to understand he was a good vet and nice to work with.

Dr. Withers was a Kansas State graduate. He was lots of fun and always kidding around. One day he came home for lunch and the phone rang. A sheet was hanging over the phone. He removed it, talked, then replaced it like he had found it. Soon the phone rang again and he removed the sheet, talked and started to replace it once more. Then he asked, "Pat, what's this sheet doing on the

The Making of a Veterinarian

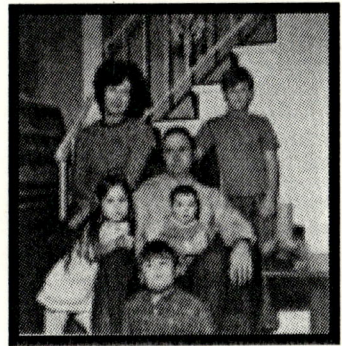
Dr. Jim Withers and family

phone?"

She said their friend Frank Korte called and told her the phone company called and said they were going to blow out the phone lines and that she might want to hang a sheet over the phone. Doc Withers really thought that was funny.

During this time at Nokomis, we increased our registered Angus cowherd from ten bred heifers to over 350 cows. We kept 100 cows at Ramsey on the Ponderosa, 100 at Bingham, and 150 out on shares. We kept weaned calves and sale bulls at Nokomis. Jesse Rogers took care of the cattle at Nokomis, Bob Snow at Bingham, and Fred Miller at the Ponderosa in Ramsey. We later sold the Ponderosa and bought more land at Bingham. We also bought forty acres from Mr. Clark at Nokomis and Lloyd Redeker helped with the cattle and Dorothy, Lloyd's wife, worked in the office.

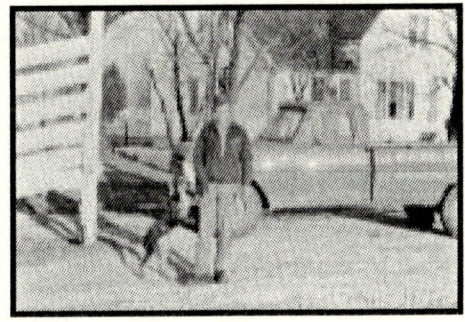
Carl Twitty, old friend and farm helper.

D.J. "Doc" McDermith

Lloyd was a fine boy and making a good hand. One day we had talked on the phone early and decided we should start raking hay when the dew dried off. I had gone on some calls, but was back in town about the time I figured the hay was ready so I ran by the field. I could just see the top of Lloyd's head at the back of the field. Then I noticed he had just raked one round and the rake was sitting about a hundred yards into the second swath.

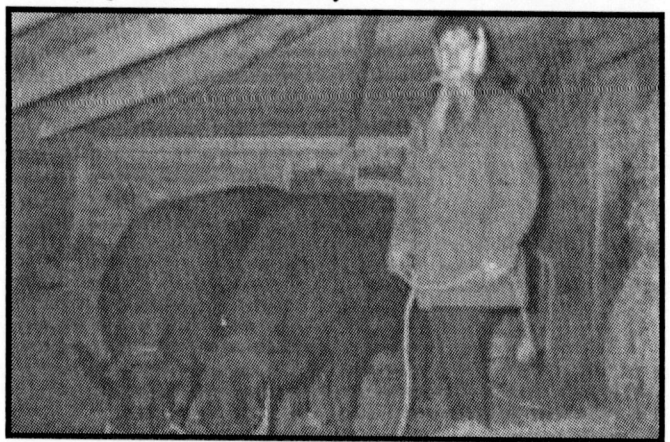

Dorothy Redeker, our veterinary office girl and Lloyd Redeker, our herdsman's wife.

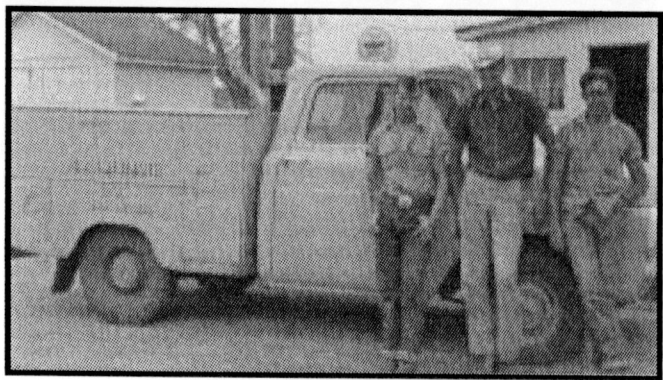

Lloyd Redeker and helpers.

The Making of a Veterinarian

I thought something must have gone wrong with our rake and maybe he had borrowed a rake from one of the neighbors. About that time he came over the hill and there was no rake on the back of the tractor. When he turned the corner and headed toward me he spied the unhitched rake. His expressions were hilarious. He looked at that rake for a few seconds then whirled around and sure enough his rake was gone. I guess that wouldn't have been so bad if I hadn't been there to see it happen.

Ben Johnson was a good friend and client. He lived in the edge of Nokomis, worked at the grain elevator and milked a few good holstein cows.

Ben's son Dennis was just starting to high school when he began coming to the clinic and going with us on calls. He decided to go to vet-school. He was the only one (out of 15 or 20 kids that thought they wanted to be veterinarians) that actually made it. Dennis originally had a general practice at Petersburgh, Illinois. He has done extensive work with accupuncture and has a small animal practice in Decatur, Illinois.

When Dennis was riding with us he would finish his lunch and go stretch out on a couch in the waiting room in the basement. One day he was on his back snoring away. His arm was sticking out to the side with his palm up. Several clients had come in, but hadn't disturbed Dennis. I squeezed his hand full of shaving cream then tickled his lip with a piece of string. He smeared shaving cream all over his face. He was afraid to go to sleep there after that. Everyone there thought it was funny, except Dennis.

D.J. "Doc" McDermith

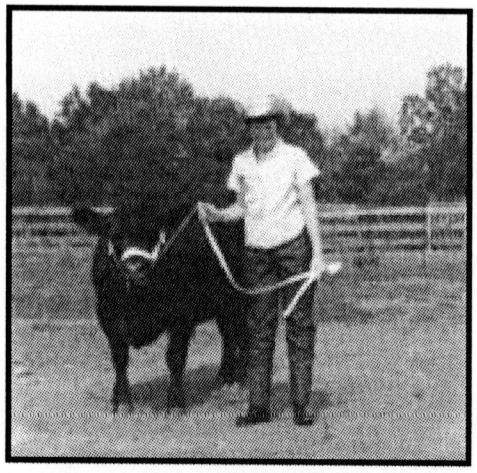

Judy Pinkston with her show heifer.

JUDY AND SUE

We lost our daughter, Carrol Ann, when she was ten days old on November 14, 1954. To make up for it, I suppose I tend to fall in love with most little girls I am around any length of time.

Blaine Pinkston, an auctioneer and one of my veterinary clients, brought his three girls over to look at some club calves. Blaine thought they were too high priced and wondered if they had diamonds in their butts, but he bought them just the same.

Judy, the middle girl, became my buddy. I would stop and take her on calls with me. She was good help and is like a daughter yet today. She married Tom Beyers and has eight beautiful children.

Probably the thing she would least want me to tell about her was when she passed out holding the instrument tray while I was spaying a cat. She was the best of help and fun to have along.

A few years later Bob Herriott and his daughters came and bought club calves. They did well in the shows and we used to see them each year at the Illinois Angus Futurity show and sale. I sold Bob more cattle for several years and Sue, his daughter, became another "adopted" daughter. She used to spend part of her school vacations with us. We have had great times trail-riding in Missouri.

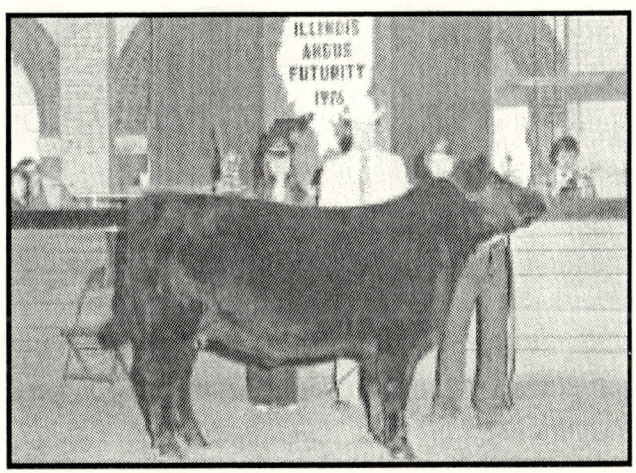

Sue Herriott showing her heifer at the Illinois Futurity Show and sale.

Sue has a great sense of humor. One evening she went with me to Birch Tree, Missouri to deliver a calf. When we drove up to the barn this little old man came out and asked us to stay in the truck until he got her in a stanchion.

He had a block of over mature fescue hay he was shaking in front of the stanchion as he said "sook, sook, sook." Sue really got a kick out of that.

Pretty soon he came out of the barn and asked if we had any grain on the truck. Sue almost blew a gasket, but she held her laughter until we started home.

Sue is an RN, has three girls, and a baby boy on the way. She is married to Jerry Henshaw, and they live near Bloomington, Illinois.

One morning about a year and a half after I started practicing, Frank Vest at Fillmore (fifteen miles south of us) called early because he had a cow down with milk fever.

While I was dressing to go, Don Large, fifteen miles north on the Taylorville black top then east about two miles, called and had one down, too. I told him I had one down at Fillmore, but would be back as soon as I could.

I had a Plymouth suburban, which would really run but was about run out. When I turned off the Taylorville blacktop heading for Don's the oil light came on.

I was getting nervous because I had a full schedule of calls from the day before these two emergencies came up. I kinda coasted to the first farmhouse on the right. I got out and checked the oil. None showed on the stick. I went to the door and knocked. A lady in a housecoat opened the door about two inches. I told her my problem, and asked if I might look in the machine shed for some oil.

She said her husband was about a half mile away in the field plowing and she was sure if he had any oil he would have it with him, and that I could drive back there and talk to him. I told her I was afraid to drive it that low on oil.

I had lived on a farm all my life and I was sure I could find some oil if she would let me look. Finally I asked her to call Don Large, that he had a cow down and maybe he could come get me. She said, "Okay! Are you the vet?" When I told her I was, she jerked that door open and said, "The can is in the machine shed and the oil is in that barrel under the tree. Help yourself!" I learned to identify myself after that.

Jesse Rogers started working for me in 1952 or '53. He was a very interesting man and very loyal to me. He lived with us like one of the family.

One evening after supper he went with me on two or three calls that were left. As we were going up a fella's lane about ten o'clock, I said I thought he had given up and gone to bed.

Jesse said, "No, I saw a light." I told him that was in the hen house. He asked why they would leave a light on in the hen house. I told him they claim they get more eggs. Jesse said, "A hen only lays one egg a day, looks like she'd have plenty time in the daylight."

One day Ed Norris, a farmer east of town, brought a sick bird dog to the clinic. He told me he had traded a

$45 fat hog for it. I kept it over night and he was to pick it up the next day.

The next day I went on a couple calls then stopped in at home. I was hitching on to my stock trailer to go pick up two registered Angus cows I had bought from my Dad. Jesse was running water in the stock tank. I asked him if he wanted to go along. He was always ready and enthusiastic to help.

I was in a hurry driving pretty fast when I noticed a farmer in the field flagging me down. As I started around the trailer to see what he wanted there was Ed's hunting dog, dead. Jesse was going to take him for a walk when he decided to let the stock tank fill up while he walked the dog. He had tied the dog to the back of the trailer and gone over in the lot to turn the water on. I drove in about that time.

I went directly to Ed's place and explained the situation. I told him how sorry I was, and that I wanted to make it right. Some animals get real expensive after they die, but Ed said he gave a fat hog worth about $45 for him. I said, "Well, the bill was $9, how would $36 sound?" He said that was fair enough. I was very sad about the whole deal but very relieved.

One evening I stopped by the house. I was on my way to test a small herd of cows and Jesse Rogers decided to go with me. The air was damp, wind blowing and really chilly and he almost froze. He said he was going to put his long underwear on that night.

The next day at noon I stopped at home for lunch.

The Making of a Veterinarian

The sun was shining, the wind had laid, and it was really warm. Jesse was grinding feed. He came out of a little granary where he had been scooping grain into the grinder. Sweat was running down his face and dripping off his nose. He said, "I'll tell you one thing, Doc. These long underwear are a success."

Jesse sold lots of cattle for me. People enjoyed visiting with him and they also enjoyed doing business with him.

We had two yearling bulls left to sell. They weren't too good, so we had agreed to take $200 apiece for them. I told Jesse we needed their pen for some weaned bull calves.

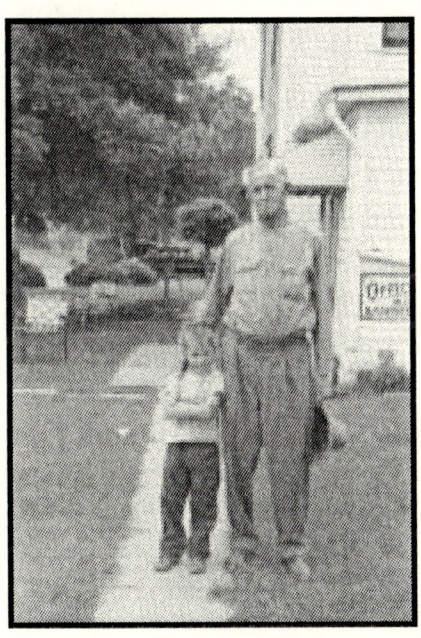

Jesse Rogers and Roger

That evening when I got home Jesse said, "I sold those bulls for $300." I was happy they were out of the way but that was below market price. Then Jesse said, "Two hundred seems awfully cheap for a bull so I told him three hundred each if he took both of them and he said, 'I'll take them.'"

D.J. "Doc" McDermith

Nancy O'Breggar stopped at the clinic one evening during office hours and was inquiring about worming her horse. I thought she should. That was before paste wormer. I advised tube worming. She wondered what that would cost if she brought her by the clinic? I told her it would be one dollar plus fifty cents per hundred. She threw her hands up beside her head and said, "Who is going to count those worms?" I meant one dollar plus fifty cents per hundred pounds the horse weighed.

About halfway between Nokomis and Fillmore lived a fellow they called "Walking Murphy." He didn't have a car and it wasn't unusual to see him on the road about any day going one way or the other. Jerry Crow, who managed Mohawk appliances in Nokomis, picked him up coming to town.

He decided to try to scare Mr. Murphy. It was a long straight stretch into Nokomis and he drove 85 and 90 all the way. When Walking Murphy got out he said, "She runs pretty good but won't hold a candle to Dr. McDermith's truck," and then walked away.

One day I made a call to a farm to assist a very small gilt that was trying to have pigs. I decided a cesarean was about the only option. I decided first to go to school and get Roger, my youngest boy, who was in the first grade and had small hands.

He was glad to get out of school, but he wasn't sure about delivering the pigs. While I was helping him roll his sleeves up and lubricate his arms he looked up at me and asked if this farmer didn't have any kids that could do this. Rog got one pig, then I gave her a shot to cause her to strain harder. Rog inserted a furacin suppository for infection and lubricant, then we left to see what she could do on her own. We found out later she did fine.

Later, we stopped at a small restaurant that was run by Mrs. Crow. She was a very nice, jolly lady. We sat down at the counter and she came to wait on us. She asked Roger if he was helping his daddy Doctor animals. He said he was and we had just doctored a sow. She said, "you mean you put pills in a sows mouth with your hand?"

Rog threw his hands up and held both sides of his head and said, "Wrong end."

She didn't ask him any more questions.

We had to do a cesarean on a big sow one day. It was six degrees below zero. The sow was in an A-house about a hundred yards from electricity. I delivered fifteen pigs and was ready to suture her up. My hands wouldn't move any more.

The farmer ran to the neighbors and got enough drop cord to get a heat light to the shed and we sutured her up. A few days later he called and said the sow was doing fine, but she had another pig. It was dead.

One day I had a call to work some cattle for Roger Smart at one of the farms he rented north of Herrick. Roger usually went in a run and was very nervous. He had done a good job of putting up a new electric fence around a clover field that I had to cross to get back where the corral was. He had pushed the wire down almost to the ground on two posts so I could drive over it. I had my cattle-working chute behind the truck so I was extra careful not to catch the wire when I drove over it.

I had an ornery idea just as I pulled up towards Roger and his hired men at the corral. I got out of the truck and instead of going toward the corral I started to the back of the trailer and asked, "Where did all that wire come from?" Roger made about three six foot circles and threw his hat on the ground. He thought I had dragged his new fence to the corral.

Ray Linder was another one of my good helpers that went with me on calls. One evening we had two Geurnsey heifers to calfhood vaccinate for a man in Nokomis. He had them in an old garden. I threw a lariat on one of them and Ray grabbed her around the neck. He said he could hold her, but instead I tied the rope to the top of a fence post with lots of slack.

When I gave her the shot she never moved, but when I tattooed her ear she threw a fit, and went completely around Ray before she got loose. The lariat was around both his legs and the heifer was running in the opposite direction from the post. Instead of stepping out of the loop he tried to take it off over his head but when the rope got to his neck it came tight.

Ray's tongue stuck out about six inches and he squalled a terrible noise. I grabbed the heifer and released the quick release Honda. Ray was in a pile on the ground rubbing his neck. I was so happy it hadn't broken his neck that I couldn't keep from laughing.

Oliver Mudd was a good horseman and a quarter

horse judge. He brought a nice quarter gelding to the clinic. They had pulled a small stick out of the muscle of his hind leg about a month before, but for some reason it wouldn't completely heal.

I told Oliver I would need to explore the wound and probably open it up some more to see if there was something else in there.

Oliver said nothing like that ever bothered him. He said he won $5 eating a sandwich sitting on a dead horse.

About that time I was enlarging the opening to the wound while Oliver was holding the horses halter. All at once I heard a big plop. Oliver had passed out and was folded up next to the horse's front legs.

We propped him against a tree, and went ahead and removed a stick about the size of a lead pencil. Oliver got some color back in about an hour, took his horse and went home.

I was removing a retained placenta from a Guernsey cow for my cousin Russell Bender, near Tower Hill. I was working away and we were visiting all the while. I happened to notice in the lot was a new born baby calf. I asked Russell if that Brahman calf was hers. He said "It is but I didn't know it was a Brahman...I noticed its ears were pretty long but I thought that was because it was born during the Democratic convention."

George DeWerff was one of my clients who had three or four milk cows on the edge of town. One of the cows was sick with indigestion. I gave her Istizin, which is a laxative and turns the urine red wine colored. It takes about twenty-four hours to work. Evidently I forgot to explain that to him. The next morning George got me out of bed. He said, "That cow ain't a bit better and she's a-pissin' blood." I explained the situation to him and everything turned out all right.

Georges's son Melvin was very conservative. We had been using calf scour pills that cost twenty cents each and we gave two the first dose then one twice daily for four days. One evening Melvin came to the clinic for some medicine for another calf that was really scouring bad.

We had just gotten some new pills that cost five dollars each. He took one and said he would get more if this one didn't take care of it.

A couple days later he called and said the calf wasn't any better. I asked when he had given the five dollar pill. He said it was so expensive he hadn't given it yet!

One Sunday morning about church time Vic Jostes had a cow down with milk fever. He said she was in a box stall in the barn and wondered if I would need him to stay home from church. I told him I was sure I could handle it. I had a hard time getting away from the office and they came home from church while I was treating the cow. Vic and his little four or five year old girl came to the barn. Vick and I visited and the little girl played in the feedway. Pretty soon there was a lull in the conversation. The little girl gave a big sigh and said, "I wonder

The Making of a Veterinarian

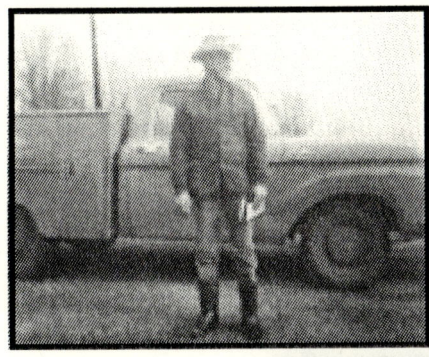

Dr. McDermith home for lunch.

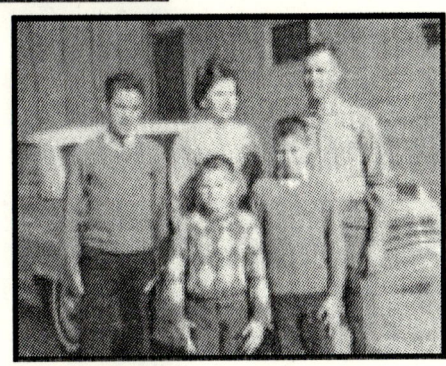

Doc, Janey and Boys at home in Nokomis.

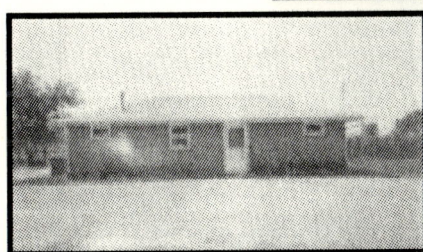

New Vet Clinic - 1959

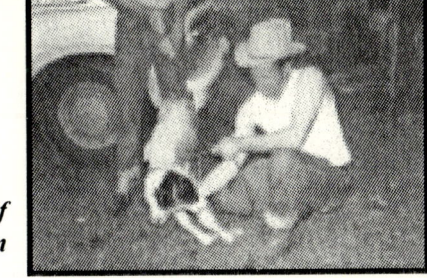

Two-headed calf delivered by Cesarean

when my mother is going to holler and tell me to come change these clean clothes."

Pee Wee (Logan Frailey), who had worked for my Dad for eight years, was helping Janey when we moved from our office in the basement to our new clinic. They had the station wagon loaded and Pee Wee was holding the typewriter. My truck was sitting near the clinic door. I had just finished office hours and as Janey was making a u-turn to back up to the clinic, I had gotten in the truck and started backing out. Neither of them had seen me get in the truck, which was moving away from the clinic. This made Janey and PeeWee feel like the station wagon hadn't stopped, and they thought they were going to hit the clinic. I saw something was wrong and stopped. They were both white as a sheet. PeeWee said his fingerprints would always be in that typewriter.

Janey was raised on a dairy farm near Oconee. She had three older brothers and two twin younger brothers. Her job after school was to fill the cattle tank with water with a hand pump. Sometimes the cows would come up and drink while she was pumping. She didn't like that because they could drink it faster than she could pump it. She would drive them away then hurry and pump the tank full. That worked until her Dad caught her.

Janey was a great partner. She practically raised our three boys with Jesse Rogers our hired man's help. She was always ready to help when the need arose.

The Making of a Veterinarian

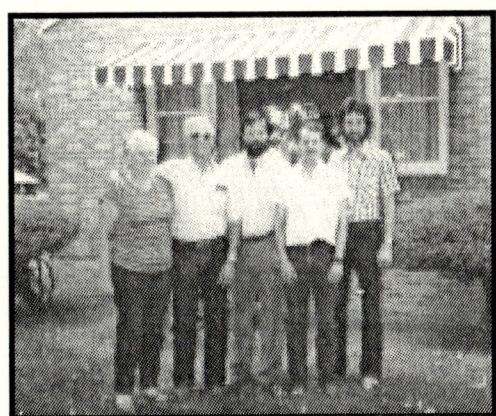

Janey, Doc, Rog, Scott and Monte

One day a client at Bayle City had a herd of Charolais beef cows break into a bean granary. He found one cow dead and several more noticeably sick and bloated. We treated twelve or thirteen with mineral oil or milk of magnesia and antihistamine.

Before I got home the farmer called the office and they called me on the two-way radio that one cow was bloated, grunting and about to go down.

We decided to do a rumenotomy and get the beans out of her rumen. When the rumen was first punctured the sour swollen beans would blow out clear across the stall. Before we finished suturing the first cow back up another one was in trouble. Before we finished her two more were in trouble. We put a trocar in one to try to keep her alive until we could operate on the other one.

By this time I realized I was short on procaine and suture. We called Janey and she rushed right out with it. Just as she stepped inside the stall door I incised the fifth cows rumen, and blew sour beans all over her. It was really funny, but I sure didn't laugh so you could notice it. We operated on eight cows. They all lived, but one cow we hadn't treated or operated on died the next night.

Many times Janey, the boys, and I would start getting our horses ready to go to a horse show or parade and before we could get them loaded and gone someone would have an emergency and I would go, leaving Janey to take the boys. We always considered our clients first, day or night.

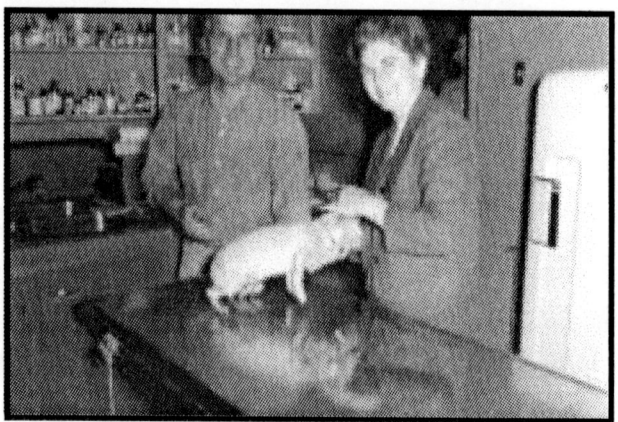

Doc and Janey trimming a Chihuahua's toenails at the new clinic.

When I got out of vet school my Dad told me to not get like bankers. He said. "People go to borrow money, no matter what for, and they want to impress the banker so they ask what he thinks about what they are buying or doing. He may know and give them some good advice, but he may not know anything about it. After so many ask him he will just tell them something. If someone asks you a question, and you know the answer, tell them. If you don't know, tell them you don't know."

Dad's banker retired and a younger man in the bank had become president. Dad went in to borrow some money. While a girl was typing up the note Dad was visiting with the banker about the Tri County fair in town, which was just over. The girl brought the note back and the banker pushed it over for Dad to sign. As he was pushing it over Dad said he was really having a problem with his wife. The banker slowly slid the note back out of Dad's reach and inquired about the problem. Dad said he brought her to town during the fair and she saw all those women wearing shoes and now she wants a pair. The banker pushed the note back and Dad signed it.

Dad had a good Angus cow that the toes on one back foot would grow out and roll to the inside. It had to be trimmed about every year and she was really crazy when you went to handle her. We had her in a big barn with two rows of posts down the middle. I roped her and handed the rope to Dad. He wrapped it twice around a square post.

I ran her back past him but she went too fast and he didn't get the slack taken up. When she hit the end, the rope jerked out of Dad's hands and went flying around the post and struck his legs just above the knees. It really hurt him. He dropped his pants down to see what it had done to his legs. They were fiery red but no blood.

Then I noticed he was getting blood all over his

pants and his little finger was almost torn off. I said, "My truck is right outside the door. We had better go get that finger sewed back on." I noticed he was getting pale and large beads of sweat were forming on his forehead. I took him by the arm and asked if he could make it to the truck.

He said, "Sure, I never did use that finger to walk with."

In the early sixties several of Dad's customers were needing beef cows and he couldn't find enough of them. One day he asked if I'd go with him to Maryville, Missouri to a cow sale. Dr. Port had worked with me five years but he had bought a practice in Athens, Illinois, and I was working day and night. I told him I couldn't go. About a month later he asked me again. I thought he might be gone one of these days and I'd wish I had gone, so I went.

Dad had a nice '59 Lincoln and he let me drive. We had a good visit going over there, but Dad thought the cows were too high. It got dark pretty quick after we started home. The road was four lane, but part of the time our side was the old highway. I was driving seventy-five and eighty. I had the lights on dim as we were meeting several cars. We came up on a curve and the tires squalled all the way around. I said, "Dad you should have those lights adjusted. They sure don't shine very far on dim."

We went a mile or two and Dad looked up and said, "I don't believe there is anything wrong with those lights. You have to give them a little time to shine."

I thought we should start looking for a motel before they were all filled up. We stopped at a new Holiday Inn. We both went in and told the clerk we needed a room. The clerk asked, "One double bed or two?"

I looked at Dad and he said he didn't care. The clerk looked at his list and said he had one with two double beds where we'd be more comfortable. "It's only a dollar more, eleven dollars."

When we walked back to the car Dad said, "He made that dollar pretty easy. One double bed is all we really need."

After Dad took his shower he said, "These are vibrating beds. I think I'll put a quarter in mine. I have trouble going to sleep when I'm away from home."

I took a shower. When I started to bed, Dad asked if I was going to put a quarter in my bed. I said I guessed I would. He said there wasn't any use, to just get in bed with him. It was real comfortable and I was almost asleep, when Dad sat up in bed and put his hand on my shoulder. He said, "Now don't you go to sleep in here or else he beat us out of that dollar." I wouldn't take anything for that trip.

Dad told me that when he was in grade school, he walked to school with several other kids. One evening they were coming home and several milk cows were out along the road. They decided to each grab one by the tail. When they did each cow took off running. They were going down hill on a gravel road. Dad's cousin Harve

Jones hung on too long. When he let loose his head was going faster than his feet and he went sliding on the gravel out into a patch of blackberry briars alongside the road. The kids ran to check on him and someone asked if he was hurt.

He said, "Hell yes I'm hurt and I'm hurt bad. We need to find out whose cows those are and have them to keep them in or they are going to kill someone!"

In the early sixties we were needing to spend some time with the boys. I had a client that built farrowing houses. He built us one with a few minor changes. We moved it to a ninety-six acre pasture with some timber and used it for a cabin.

Paul Mudd, my vet helper, built bunk beds and Janey gathered up utensils to cook on an open fire. It was great to get away from the phone and the work.

We camped with friends, like the Clifford and Dorothy Betzold family, the trail riders, and church people. As I look back we probably should have done a lot more of that.

I think one of Janey's greatest accomplishments was getting Clifford to sell his Hereford cows and buy Angus from us.

I had 90 Angus cows. Clifford wanted to pick 30 head. I told him I would pick 30 that he couldn't have, then he could pick 30 from the 60 that were left and we made a deal.

Janey and Clifford were always arguing whether Hereford or Angus cattle were the best. After that they

The Making of a Veterinarian

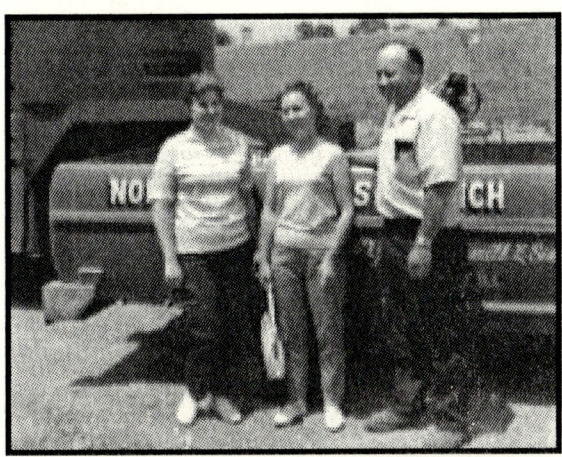

Janey with Dorothy and Clifford Betzold, our very close friends.

didn't have anything left to argue about.

Clifford was pretty good to bite on my jokes, but he finally wouldn't believe anything I told him. He really laughed when I told him President Kennedy had been shot and he wouldn't believe a word of it.

Merrill Sorrells, Dorothy Betzold's father, had a trucking business and farm supply in Raymond, Illinois, and his son Earl managed the family farm. Merrill and I got off to a rocky start. He called on December 31 at noon and wanted 155 pigs castrated and vaccinated for Cholera and Erysipelas. I told him we had done a large bunch that morning and I only had 60 doses of Cholera, but I could have it the next morning. We were supposed to be there at 8 a.m.

The next morning a helper, a friend and I were on

our way to his place when we got a call about a cow having trouble calving. I didn't take time to call him and we got there about 30 minutes late. Earl and two hired men and my two helpers went to the barn to pin the pigs. I explained to Merrill why we were late and thought that would be sufficient. Merrill asked, "Was that cow booked ahead of me?"

I told him, "No, but we have to take care of emergencies first."

He said, "If that's the way you run your business, I'll get someone else next time."

Then I asked him, "Do you still want us to do these pigs?"

He said, "Yes, while you're here."

When we finished the pigs he made arrangements to dehorn his cows, and castrate, dehorn, and vaccinate the calves.

Merrill and Earl were great friends of ours and sent lots of business my way. Earl and Doris took Janey and I to our first International Livestock Exposition in Chicago and also to the Museum of Arts and Sciences. We had many great times together.

One night I was coming home past Earl's farm and a light was still on in the house. I pulled in and visited with them a few minutes. When I started back to the truck Doris and Earl both came out on the porch and pulled the door shut. They had already locked the doors for the night, so they were locked out.

Earl and I finally pushed Doris up on top of the

back porch and she got in the window of their daughter, Brenda's bedroom. The next morning Brenda asked Doris, "Did you come in my window last night, or was I dreaming?"

In 1970 I started at seven each morning, and often worked until one or two-o-clock the next morning. We were booked so far ahead that it was almost impossible to get away to relax. I was having trouble with my back, which wasn't serious but annoying. I would get to the office, the phone would be ringing, and people would be at the office to catch us before we got away.

Our call book, which held twenty-five calls, would be full and some in the margins. Usually four or five of those calls were emergencies that had to be made before we started on our days work.

I had good help; Mrs. Robb was in the office and Tom Stokes was on the truck. Janey kept books and sent out the bills besides lots of other odd jobs in a pinch.

All at once I started getting sick at my stomach and very nervous before I could get away from the office in the morning. When we finished with emergencies and started on our planned days work I would start feeling fine and would work to all hours of the night until everything was done. I decided life was too short to live like that and I had a cattle operation that I thought would support me with lots less work and stress.

Dr. Lacey was interested in my practice, so I made him a proposition. He was going home that weekend and said he would let me know Monday. When he came back he said he would rather work for me a year and then buy it. I told him he wasn't going to work for me a year because I didn't think I would last a year, so he went ahead and bought it. He married Ruth Ann Smith, one of my little girl friends, raised a great family (Roquel and Hunt) besides serving the people well in his practice.

Ten businessmen, including myself, built and directed the Nokomis Golden Manor Nursing home in Nokomis, Illinois until we sold it after several years. It was originally 49 units and we added another 25 units over the next couple of years. It was and still is a great asset to the community.

SHELLABARGER FARM 1970-1976

I was delivering pigs for Rufus Niermi, a realtor, and told him I would be selling my place in Nokomis within the next year. I was planning to build a new home at Bingham place. Within a week he sold it.

A few days later I was delivering pigs for Cliff Shellaberger. He had a new home on twenty acres a mile south of Ramsey. He said why don't you buy this farm so I can move to Arizona where my daughter lives. That interested me because I was really dreading building a home. I took Janey to see it and she liked it so we bought it.

This farm worked great. It took the place of the Nokomis farm. It was a good place to show our sale bulls and a good place to wean our calves. We would weigh and grade the calves, castrate the lower half of the bulls and cull a few heifers. We sorted the bulls off to develop for herd bulls to sell. The good heifers were separated and developed for cows, or sold for club calves.

D.J. "Doc" McDermith

A hundred head of cows needs about fifteen heifers to replace old cows and culls. The lower end of the steers and heifers are straightened up over weaning, given their shots, and taught to eat out of a bunk and then they're sold for stockers around 500#. If we had plenty of feed and grass we might keep them to seven or eight hundred pounds, and sell them for feeders, where they would go directly to the feedlot.

I had promised Dr. Lacey I would work for him three days a week for a year. With what I was trying to do on the farm and helping Dr. Lacey I was pretty busy, but it was a great deal better than when I was practicing by myself.

We had sold the ninety-six acres on the county line, hog house cabin and all, and bought the Ponderosa about one mile east of Ramsey. We were enjoying the old farmhouse as a get away and entertained lots of our friends there. It was the Miller farm where Fred Miller, who looked after the cows there, was raised. It started out a hundred and forty-seven acres. We kept adding to it, the John Cashin place, Kirkpatrick's, Pasley, until it was over two hundred and fifty acres. We built a twenty by sixty concrete silo and auger bunk.

When we were building the bunk, I told Rog to hurry home from school. I wanted him to help me finish it that evening. Rog was good help but he didn't hurry and I was pushing him pretty hard. He backed up the tractor with post auger to drill the last two holes. I grabbed the auger to put it on the spot. He turned the power take off on before I turned loose. The corner of the auger caught my new leather glove and jerked my arm completely around the auger, and my neck against the power take off. I thought my time had come.

All at once my glove split and turned me loose. Rog froze and I turned the auger off. We finished the bunk but I had a pretty sore arm and neck the next morning.

We had a chance to buy more land adjoining the Bingham farm so we wouldn't have to be running back and forth so much with the machinery. We sold the ponderosa to Dr. Coulter and Ronnie Stapp who raised Chianina cattle.

We built a twenty by sixty concrete silo for corn silage and a twenty-five by eighty harvestore for grass silage at Bingham. The harvestore really kept us busy through the summer trying to fill it.

One morning my oldest boy Monte climbed the harvestore. It was filled up to two and a half rings from the top, twelve and a half feet. We had a good day and put eighteen, six-ton loads of grass silage in. Monte climbed to the top again with a flashlight and he was really discouraged to find out it was three rings or fifteen feet from the top. The silage eventually quit settling and we finally got it full.

Things were going good. I wasn't doing vet work any more, except my own. Monte and Rog were helping me.

Monte was married to Marsha Hortensteine and

they had Holly and Josh. Monte and Marsha later divorced, and he married Robin Goodman and together they had Jessica. Monte managed a fertilizer plant in southern Illinois for a few years. He then started a plant of his own in Ramsey. Later he drove a truck until he became disabled with congenital Myotonic Dystrophy.

Rog married Paula Werner and had Dusty. Rog worked in construction for awhile. Later he bought his own 18-wheeler and trucked until he became disabled as well. He now lives independantly in his home in Vandalia, Illinois.

Scott married Debbie Redman and they had Joni. They divorced and he married Marla Childers and had Rhianna. Scott worked in factories in Vandalia and Effingham. He also fell victim to Myotonic Dystrophy. He lives with his daughter, Joni, and grandkids in Effingham, Illinois.

Having lost our only daughter Carrol Ann in 1954 when she was ten days old, our daughters-in-law were very special to us, especially Paula. She and Rog lived in our basement for a while after they were married. She was so sweet, yet mischievous.

One evening she was running the sweeper in the living room. The electric cord scooted a pan of popcorn off the coffee table and spilled it all over the floor. She got the broom and dustpan, swept it up and put it back in the pan and set it back on the coffee table. Paula went on vacuuming in other parts of the house. I came in starved for supper, turned on the TV and started eating the popcorn. Paula finally came to throw out the dirty popcorn and it was all gone. She really thought that was funny.

When Dusty was about nine months old, Janey and I thought he and Paula were about the greatest thing in our lives. Rog had bought a double-wide trailer and set it up on the farm at Bingham, next to a pond. Paula was mowing the grass around it one evening. I told her not to run that lawnmower into the pond. I told her I didn't care so much about her, but I didn't want her to ruin my new lawn mower. I'll never forget the look she gave me. That was the last time I saw her alive.

I didn't know it at the time but that evening they ate supper at their trailer they rented in Ramsey, then went to the new trailer and slept on the floors. After Rog left the next morning, Paula went to the old trailer and loaded some stuff to take to the new trailer. Dusty was with her in the front seat asleep. It was just starting to sprinkle. They were going downhill around a curve when the car skidded out of control and into the path of a loaded grain semi-truck. They were both killed. I wished it had been me, and I'm sure Janey felt that way too. I never had a pain like that before or since.

Rog never did move into the trailer. This was in October and the next April a tornado scattered the trailer and all of Paula and Dusty's belongings over forty acres. People came from all around and helped us gather stuff up and get it in to dry.

We could handle about two hundred cows at Bingham. I decided to bring the cows that were out on

D.J. "Doc" McDermith

shares home. The person keeping the cows and I divided the calves fifty-fifty. I also furnished the bulls and vet service. It had worked well, but I needed to slow down and I enjoyed having all of them under our care.

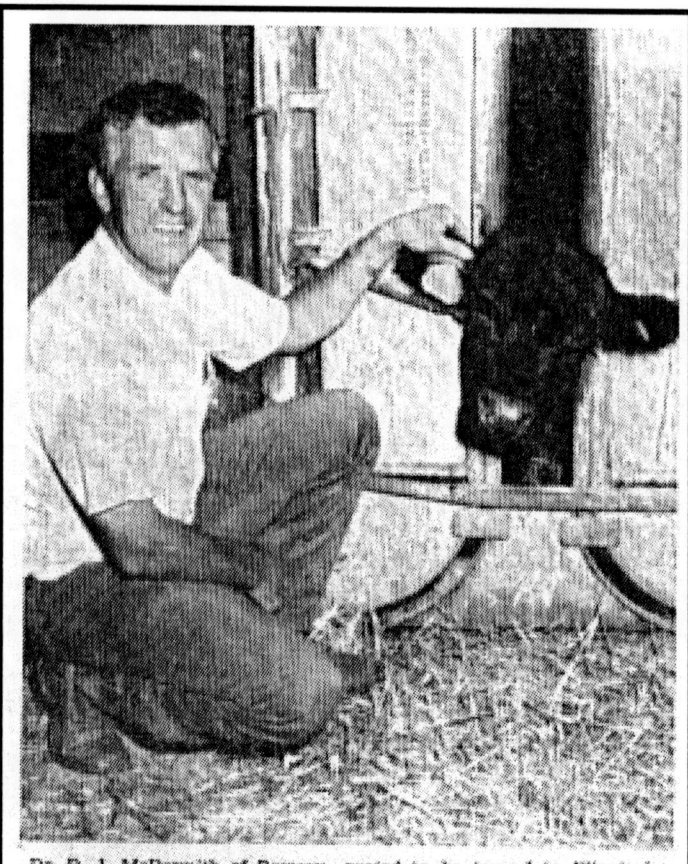

Dr. D. J. McDermith of Ramsey, formerly of Nokomis, is the first beef producer in the nation to ear tag a calf going to market for which he wants an evaluation of the quality and cutability of the carcass. About 2,500 calves are expected to be tagged in Illinois by next fall. Prospects for success of the new cooperative carcass data reporting program are termed as excellent. The beef was tagged Wednesday at the McDermith farm. —Nokomis Free Press-Progress

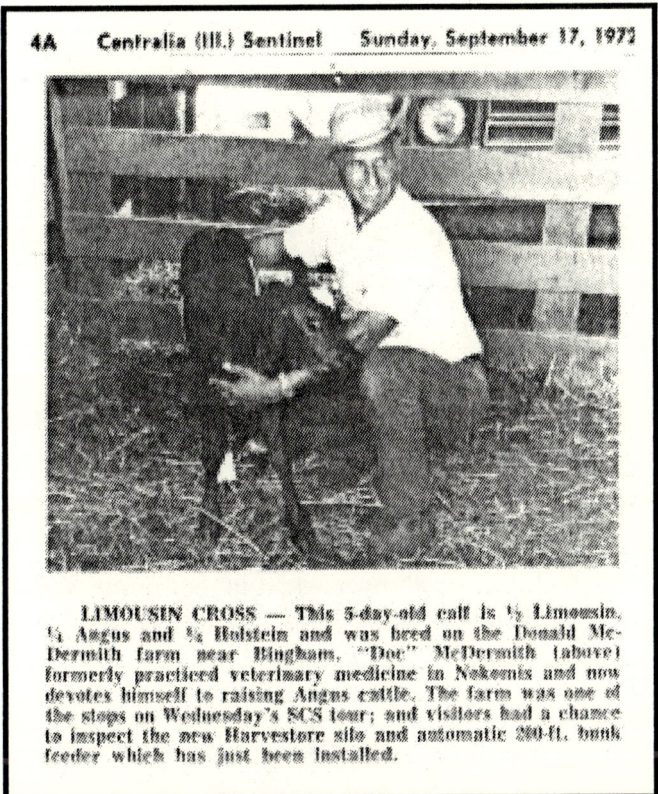

One day I was getting my hair cut in Vandalia and the real-estate man next door, Mr. Bunyard, stopped and asked me if I would sell the Bingham farm. I didn't price it, but the next time I got my haircut I priced it and within a week he sold it to a coal company that was trading it for another farm.

I rented five hundred acres of pasture from Hunt Taylor for a couple of years. He was great to rent from.

He and Janey would team up against me and give me a rough time. I wasn't satisfied without owning my own place.

The sale barn at Greenville sent me a livestock paper for years. One month there was a fifteen hundred acre ranch at Alton, Missouri that sounded interesting. I talked my Dad and Roger Smart, an auctioneer at Herrick, Illinois, into coming with me. We looked at that farm and a few others but none really suited. Then something pretty funny happened.

We left home before daylight. We were nearing St. Louis and Dad needed to urinate so we stopped at a station. Roger Smart and I waited and waited until finally Dad came out. We inquired what the problem was. He said he had taken a shower when he got up, it was still dark and he got his shorts on backwards. He had to take his pants and boots off so he could turn his shorts around. Roger laughed for fifty miles. That was in April.

In June I had a registered Angus sale and sold seventy-nine cows. By that time every real estate person in Southern Missouri knew I wanted a cow ranch and I got brochures every week, so after the sale I went back by myself. The third day I found just what I wanted, the Bob Smith or Dankert five hundred forty-seven acres, nice home, machine shed, and new barn, north of Summersville, Missouri. We bought hay and all, and took possession the first of November. Dad and Janey really liked the place, which really made me happy.

Rog was working on construction and had bought

Sam Beck's farm about three miles north of Ramsey on Highway fifty-one.

Soon after Rog moved to the farm, he had a streak of bad luck. The wiring caught the house on fire and he was almost asphyxiated before he woke up.

Then some of his cattle got a wire gap down at two a.m. and got out on the highway. A trailer truck hit and killed five of them and a car hit the back of the truck. Three of the calves were half mine.

The people in the car sued Rog for $500,000. He only had $25,000 insurance. Rog kept the farm for three years, but it took five years for the court to decide that my insurance and the truck insurance were partly liable. The seventh year they settled with the people for $87,000.

D.J. "Doc" McDermith

BOB SMITH (DANKERT PLACE)
NOVEMBER 1976 TO NOVEMBER 1977

Ten friends helped us move to Missouri. It was almost evening when we got eleven trucks loaded in Illinois, and it was eleven that night when we got to the farm in Summersville. We had wall-to-wall guests that night. We knew no one in the area, but we had lived with hired help for so many years we were kinda glad to be alone.

It was a hard winter with lots of snow and we hadn't burned wood for years. We cleaned up a bunch of dead fruit trees and burned the wood early while it was warm. Every time we made a fire it almost ran us out of the house, then when it really got cold we were cutting green wood and it would sizzle while we were freezing.

There was a great big oak tree that had died about a quarter mile from the house that I decided I would cut down. I cut all the way around it and notched it, but it wouldn't fall. I finally borrowed some wedges from my neighbor Homer Smith and got it to fall.

We fed the cows two pounds of cubes every morning. There was about a foot of snow on and it was around zero. We had a big pond that was completely surrounded by trees. I looked all over the cleared pasture and the cows weren't in sight. We drove into the wooded area and there, bedded down on the pond, were 79 cows.

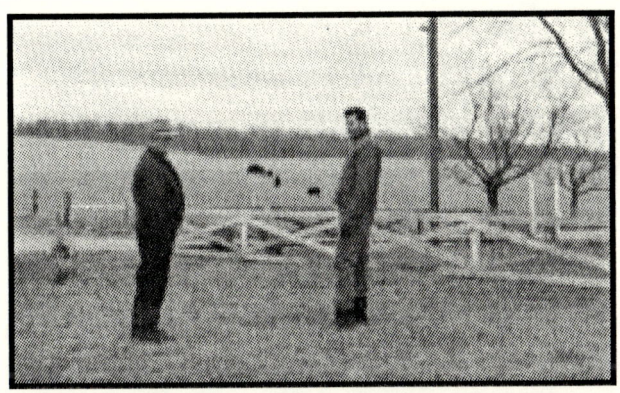

Dad and Kenneth Casey down from Illinois after we sold out to Kenneth.

I couldn't believe they hadn't broken through the ice. Quickly, we started feeding the cubes and calling them off the ice. I built a fence around the pond that same day.

One Sunday, after it had warmed up some, Homer Smith and I were on that pond for some reason. The ice was mixed with snow and mostly white, but there were spots about eight or ten inches across that were clear. I asked Homer if he knew what caused that. I had tried to break it with my heel several times.

About that time, I tried once more. It broke through and I went in, up to my straddle. I could hardly get my foot out and my boot was full of water. Homer laughed and laughed that day and laughed more anytime it was mentioned later.

We hadn't planned to do any vet work down here in Missouri. We just aimed to raise registered Angus cattle.

We helped Homer work his cattle and had a great time together riding horses and going places together. Homer knew everyone and introduced us to everyone he knew. Ethel, Homer's wife, made good biscuits and laughed at my jokes. They always included us in their family gatherings, which we really enjoyed and appreciated.

Before the year was over I sold the place to Kenneth and Verla Casey, friends and clients from Vandalia, Illinois.

I had worked up and resowed a field of grass and it looked great. Dad was here on a visit and said that it would be nice to own a field of grass like that. He was kidding me because I had sold it.

The Making of a Veterinarian

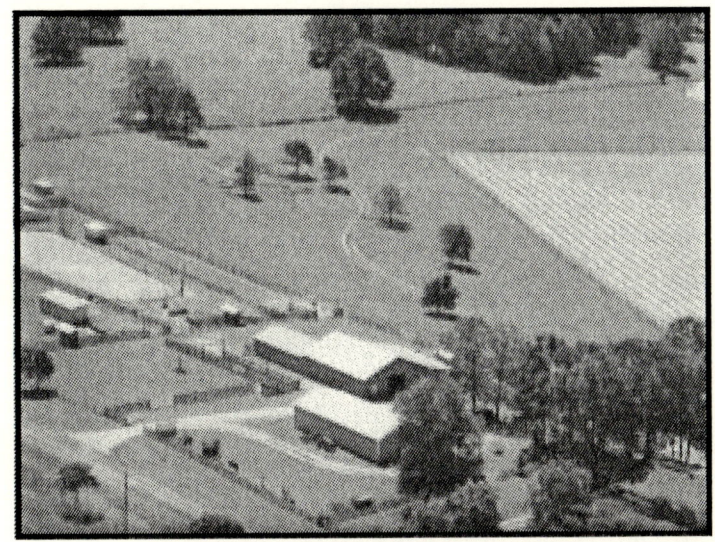

JERRY GILES PLACE
NOVEMBER 1977 TO MAY 1996

When we moved to the Giles place near Summersville there were lots of sprouts, the fences were in need of repair and the soil was run down. We had three registered quarter horse mares, a stud, 150 registered cows, and we bought 200 goats to help on the sprouts.

More people kept calling wanting us to do large animal vet work. Finally we bought another pick up and a vet bed for it. That was a mistake because our vet work really picked up then.

We rented another eighty acres from Edgar Allen and eighty acres from my boy Rog. Rog had quit working on construction in 1979 and moved to Missouri with us. He bought eighty acres on K highway and we rented it from him. He helped out and cut cordwood with Gregg Wilcox. Roger went to SMSU in Springfield for a year.

We built our brood mares up to eighteen and dispersed them in 1984. We were enjoying the Saddle Club and trail rides so much that we bought a couple of gaited horses.

The goats did a good job in the sprayed timber and small sprouts but we had seventy acres where the sprouts were ten or twelve feet tall that the goats couldn't handle even though they did help a lot. We still had to doze it off, and sow it with fescue.

In 1979 I went to Fillmore, Illinois and bought red clover seed from Curtis Hopwod. My plan was to establish clover in our fescue and orchard grass pastures, which would improve the quality of pasture and hay.

Clover produces nitrogen that can be utilized by the grass, reducing the need for much nitrogen in the fertilizer, which is the highest priced ingredient. We main-

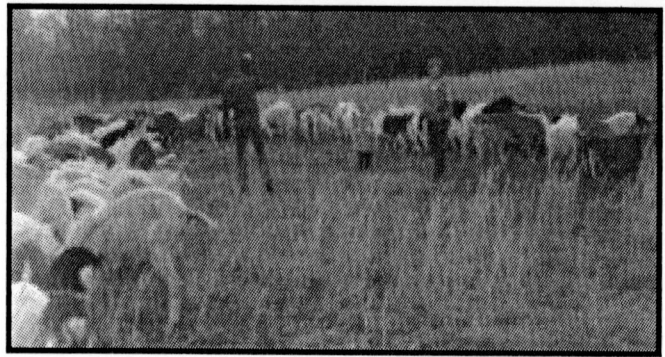

Janey, Monte and Jessi watching the goats eat.

The Making of a Veterinarian

McDermith Appointed To Beef Committee

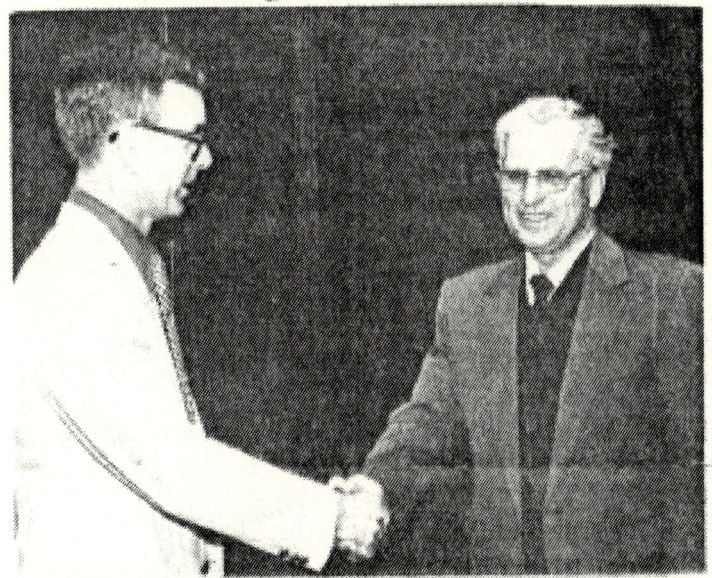

Dr. Don McDermith of Summersville, Mo. has been appointed to the Missouri Farm Bureau Beef Advisory Committee. The committee held its first meeting at the Missouri Farm Bureau Center in Jefferson City, January 4 and 5.

The committee studies state and federal regulations affecting the beef industry as well as issues of concern to the cattle industry. The committee then makes policy recommendations to the Missouri Farm Bureau State Resolutions Committee. The committee also works closely with the Missouri Cattlemen's Association in the promotion of beef products.

During the two-day meeting, the committee members met with Al Keating, Director of the Livestock Department at the American Farm Bureau Federation; Ron Morrow, of the Animal Science Department at the University of Missouri; Russell Harriman, Executive Secretary of the Missouri Cattlemen's Association; Dr. Ed Slauter, Director of Animal Health at the Missouri Department of Agriculture and Steve Carpenter, Director of Market Development at the Missouri Department of Agriculture.

McDermith has a 480 acre farm on which he raises registered Angus cows and quarter horse brood mares.

tained a good stand by mixing three or four pounds of clover seed in the fertilizer every year. If you include too much nitrogen in the fertilizer it will overstimulate the grass and crowd out the clover.

In the late 1980's I planted about twenty-five acres of a Russian warm season grass called Caucasian Blue Stem. It was of high quality and very productive, but

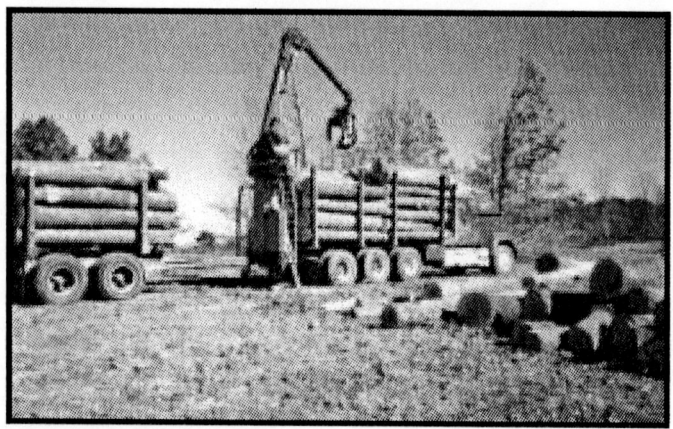

Ronnie Harper clearing 165 scattered trees on the Giles place (60 acre pasture).

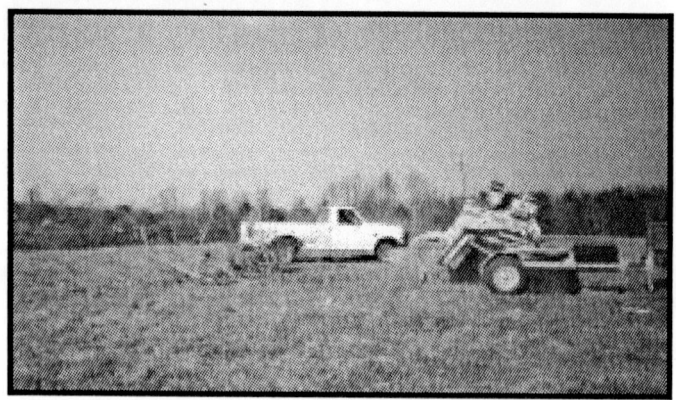

Frank Miller from Success, MO grinding the 165 stumps out.

required lots of management. It helped to burn it off about the first of May to get rid of cool season competition. Fertilizer needs to be put on about June first, when the grass is ready to start growing. A registered Angus herd was maintained for forty-six years while practicing veterinary medicine 22 years at Nokomis, Illinois, then twenty more years at Summersville, Missouri. In Mis-

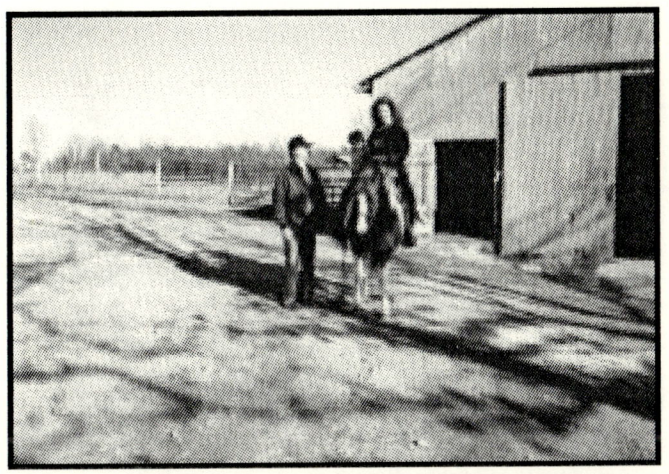

Granddaughters Joni and Rhianna taking a ride.

souri we also kept from ten to eighteen quarter horse brood mares for seven or eight years. We fed cattle continuously for seven or eight years in a feedlot at Oconto, Nebraska.

Dad always said he would never fly in a plane, but in 1981, when he was eighty years old, we talked Dad and Mom into meeting us in St. Louis and flying to California to visit Jim's family in San Bernadino, and Sis's family in Livermore. When we got up and leveled out, I asked how he liked flying. He said, "I knew I would enjoy flying, it was if it *didn't* fly that I was worried about."

I had open heart surgery in 1985. The work, book work and vet work was getting to be too much for Janey, (and me too) so we advertised our Registered Cows and sold them to a man in Oklahoma in 1987. After selling the cows I decided to buy eighty or ninety, four hundred pound, black or black baldy heifers and develop them for

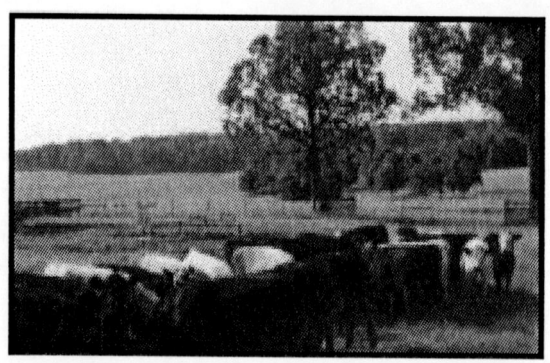

Angus and Angus Cross heifers being developed for mother cows.

cows. We wormed them, calfhood vaccinated them for brucellosis, seven-way blackleg, vibriosis and five strains of lepto, as well as the respiratory viruses. We used several different forms of fly control at different times and then when they weighed seven or eight hundred pounds and were fourteen to sixteen months old we bred them to easy calving bulls for sixty days. Then we waited another sixty days, pregnancy tested them and checked pelvic measurement and for deformities of the pelvis. We ad-

The Making of a Veterinarian

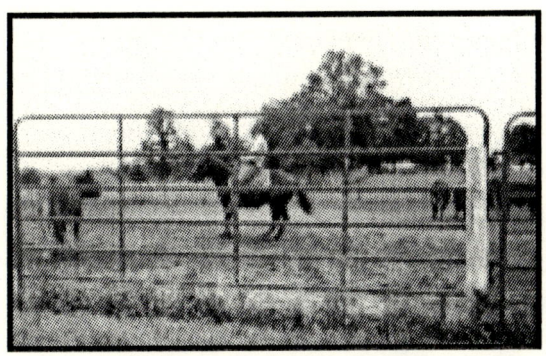

Burl Jones training "Peppy".

vertised the bred heifers and sent the open ones to the sale barn. We developed two batches a year for nine more years.

In the spring of '86 I went to Salem, Arkansas to a horse sale and bought a yearling quarter colt bred to be a cutting horse. His name was San Peppy Doc and we called him "Peppy." We decided to have Burl Jones at Koshkonong, Missouri train him. Peppy placed second in the Missouri Futurity and made the finals at the Kansas Futurity. I kept him several years and he was a great enjoyment. Later, I sold him to a rancher at Rolla, Missouri. Peppy lost money, but I loved every minute of it.

One Saturday Ronnie Smith, Homer's son, helped me work on horses all day. We were planning to eat at his house that evening. I had told him a weld in my field roller was cracked and leaking water. We came home to do my chores in the evening and Ronnie said if I would back that roller in the shed he would weld it while I fed. When I finished feeding he was still welding and with the hood on he hadn't noticed me walk up. I slipped in the shop and got a sledge hammer and hit the metal roller as hard as I could. Ronnie almost had a runaway and he was sure it had blown up. I guess he forgave me. We are still buddies.

Ronnie and Gail Smith's youngest boy Dusty went with me on a call one day when he was about three years old. He was standing in the seat beside me and I was showing him how I could wiggle my ears. He never said a word. We went another four or five miles and he tapped me on the shoulder. He had his bottom lip turned wrong side out. He could turn it back and forth without touching it. He showed me he had talent too!

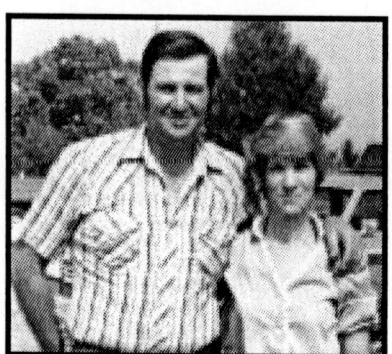
Ron and Gail Smith in 1983

Pete and Janice Howell live down on Big Creek, north of Summersville, and they both work away from home. Pete had asked me about his horse that had been biting at its flanks. I told him I didn't know why he did it unless he was bored but I would try to find out.

After Pete went to work one morning Janice noticed a cow had calved and hadn't shed the placenta. Janice called and wanted me to leave a sleeve and uterine boluses at Hodnett's station in town, which I did.

Pete was driving by Hodnett's that evening coming home from work and they flagged him down and gave him the cow medicine. In a little while Janice came by to pick up the cow medicine. When she found out what happened she said Pete would think that was for his horse.

Janice hurried home but sure enough Pete had crushed the three big uterine boluses and fed them to his horse in his feed. Pete said, "I wondered why he put them in that plastic sleeve." I thought the urea in the boluses might poison the horse, but there seemed to be no ill effects.

Frankie Shoults has a general store in Hartshorn, Missouri and also has some farms. One day he called about a sick cow. I stopped at the store to find out where the cow was and Frankie sent a boy with me to run her in the chute. When we got there I could see she had hardware (traumatic pericarditis) and was past treating. I also noticed she had a new tag number in her ear and the other cows were newly tagged.

We went back to the store and I explained the situation to Frankie. I asked him if he had a list of his cows. He scratched around under the counter and came up with it. I said if you can find her number, just draw a line through it. Frankie said, "Shore, that will work."

One evening about nine o'clock, Ralph Cooley called. He had found a cow with a newborn calf and it had a broken leg. He wanted me to wait until morning because it was down in the pasture.

I went out early the next morning. I could hear a

tractor coming up behind the barn. Ralph was on the tractor and his brother Bill was on a tote-all behind holding a newborn calf. I could see Bill was going to turn it loose in the corral. I told him to hold on a minute and I'd give it a shot. When he turned the calf loose, it just trotted off so I knew I had given the anesthesia shot to the wrong calf.

Bill and Ralph laughed for fifteen minutes before I could find out that the calf with the broken leg was still in the pasture. I called that evening to find out how the calves were doing. Ralph said the one with the broken leg was up doing fine, but the other one was still asleep. It woke up by the next morning

One day I went to Gwynn and Danny Ross's farm to pregnancy check two mares. Gwynn and Gina (their 10 or 11 year old daughter) were helping. Gina had a short haircut and a cap on. I said, "Son, if you would get on the other side of the petition and hold her tail it would sure help."

She looked at me very seriously and said, "I'll do it but I'm not a boy."

One weekend our saddle club was having a trail ride. Leslie Howell was probably about eight or nine years old. She asked me if I would hold her horse until she got on. She was a little chubby and the horse was pretty tall. I said I thought she could get on easier if she wasn't so fat.

She stopped, looked up at me and said, "You're not so skinny yourself."

When our youngest son Roger was going to SMS, he brought a friend home with him that was from Boston one weekend. Rog was going to ride his horse, Bart. He was brushing the dirt off of him and Roger's friend wanted to walk between Bart and the wall...

Rog said "That's Okay, come on through, just speak to him first."

The young man sidled behind him and said, "Hello."

Rog couldn't hardly saddle his horse for laughing.

Our oldest son Monte died from lung cancer May 16, 1994. He had been being treated for a pinched sciatic nerve for several weeks when they discovered another problem. He died 16 days after being diagnosed with lung and bone cancer.

D.J. "Doc" McDermith

THURMAN SYKES PLACE
MAY 1996

Janey was diagnosed with cancer in 1995. She had to have surgery and chemotherapy which seemed to cure her. I was having some heart problems again so we decided to sell out and move to town. We sold the last heifers in December 1995, had a farm sale in April '96, and sold the farm in May '96 to Ernest Smith, another of Homer's sons.

In May of 1996, just before selling our farm, we bought a nice home with six acres from Thurman Sykes. It had a nice garage and shop, small machine shed and another tin shed. We wanted to keep two horses so we built a tack room and hay room on the tin shed, made two horse stalls and two alleyways to park our sixteen foot horse trailer and our thirty foot horse trailer with living quarters.

We didn't get to ride much. Janey's cancer showed up again and she passed away September 20, 1997.

We brought an old blue healer named Blue that had been so much help on the farm to town with us. She and the horses were lots of comfort after Janey died.

I had never cooked and did very little house work, but I learned slowly. Riverways Hospice from West Plains took care of Janey the last few months. Several different nurses and other staff had visited her. It was soon easy to see the one she preferred and trusted the most was Barkha.

Jerri-Anne Barkha Bullin lived near Mountain View, Missouri along the Jacks Fork River. Her folks and nineteen-year-old son Shay live in North Carolina. Barkha had spent about ten years nursing in hospitals and hospices in St. Louis, Missouri before coming to the Ozarks. She was an RN for Riverways Hospice at West Plains, Missouri for four years, then in November 2001 she changed to Community Hospices of America at Mountain Grove, where she is a clinical supervisor. She also teaches yoga here in Summersville.

After Janey was gone I wanted to keep in touch with Barkha because Janey and I had appreciated her so much. I would call her occasionally. We went trail riding a few times and would sometimes go out to eat. I really enjoyed her company.

She knew about so many things I didn't, and I knew about a few things she didn't. We enjoyed explaining them to one another. We also had a lot of comparing human and animal disease processes and treatment.

She is a mushroom hunter, knows lots of them and has books to identify the ones she doesn't. There are hundreds of them. I didn't know there were over two or three kinds.

We both knew we could only be friends because there was thirty-three years difference in our age, but that changed over time. One Sunday morning I went to church. I don't remember anything about the sermon, but several things my pastor, Scott Lindsley, said made me feel like I should ask Barkha to marry me.

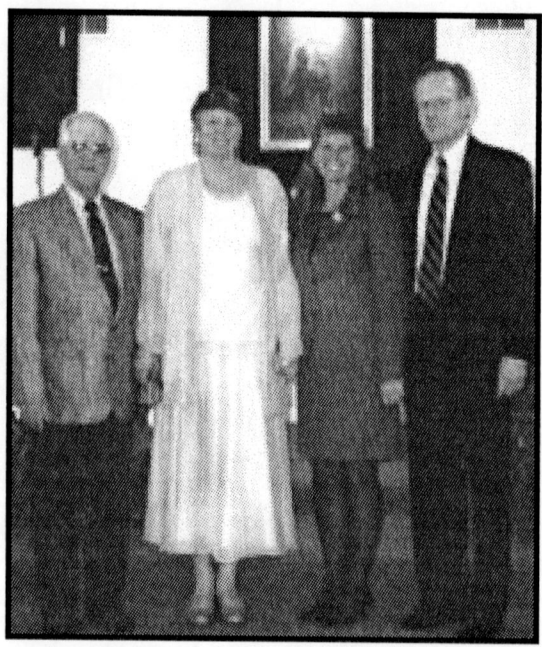

Doc and Barkha at their wedding with Sue and Jerry Henshaw.

I drove over to her house after church. She was stacking wood and cleaning up her yard. She was sweaty and dirty. I stopped the car close to her and said, "Before I forget, would you marry me?"

She said, "yes." And gave me a big old hug.

*****

We just had our second anniversary and it hasn't always been easy for either of us. The age difference hasn't been as much a problem as the way we were raised...I'm strictly country and she has spent most of her life in the city or suburbs, which causes us to look at some things differently. She enjoys the outdoors and nature. I think we are both understanding each other better each day, and I'm sure if we both keep trying everything will work out fine. We go to church, hunt mushrooms, or ride horses in her free time.

My dog Blue got killed on the highway in July of 2000. We still have Barkha's dog, Crow, a house cat, Meera, two barn cats, Tom and Tino, a Tennessee Walking horse, Billy, and a Missouri Fox Trotter, Jesse, which Barkha named after my Dad.

When we got married I told Barkha I didn't want a cat in the house. We compromised and the cat stays in the house.

D.J. "Doc" McDermith

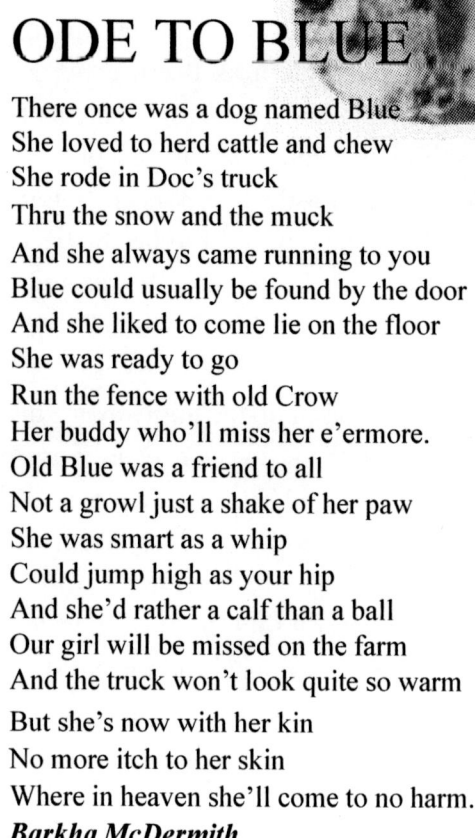

ODE TO BLUE

There once was a dog named Blue
She loved to herd cattle and chew
She rode in Doc's truck
Thru the snow and the muck
And she always came running to you

Blue could usually be found by the door
And she liked to come lie on the floor
She was ready to go
Run the fence with old Crow
Her buddy who'll miss her e'ermore.

Old Blue was a friend to all
Not a growl just a shake of her paw
She was smart as a whip
Could jump high as your hip
And she'd rather a calf than a ball

Our girl will be missed on the farm
And the truck won't look quite so warm
But she's now with her kin
No more itch to her skin
Where in heaven she'll come to no harm.
Barkha McDermith

The Making of a Veterinarian

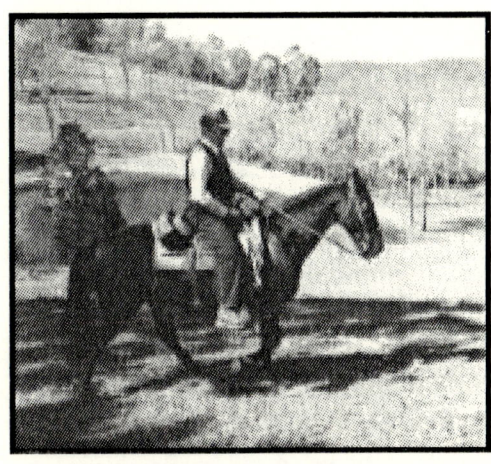

Doc coming in off a ride at Big Creek Trail Ride.

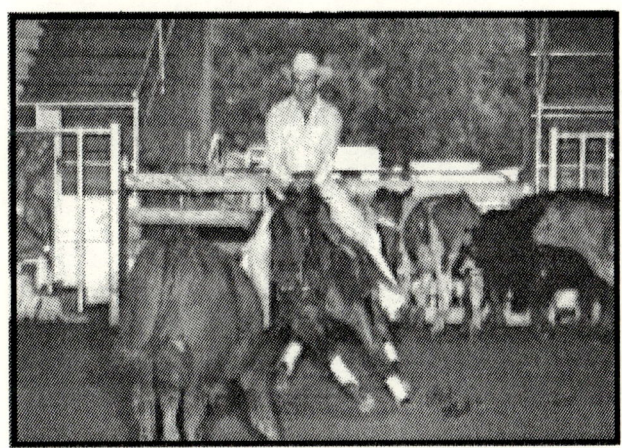

Burl Jones on "San Peppy Doc".

D.J. "Doc" McDermith

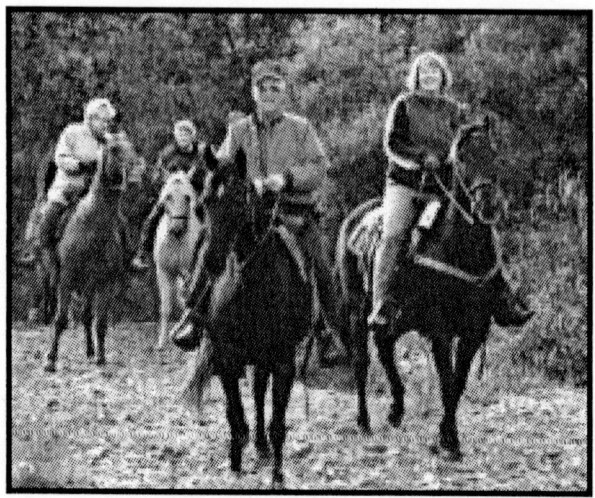

Doc and Barkha trail riding at Big Creek Trail Ride along Big Creek and Current River.

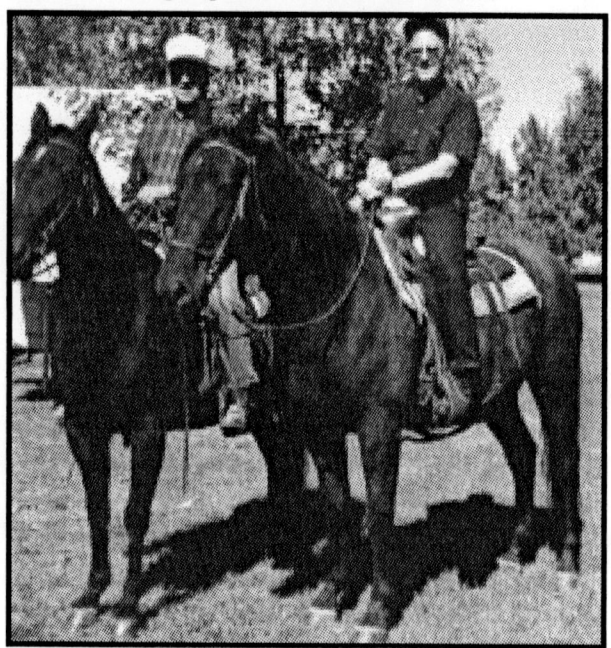

Brother Jim and Doc taking a ride.

The Making of a Veterinarian

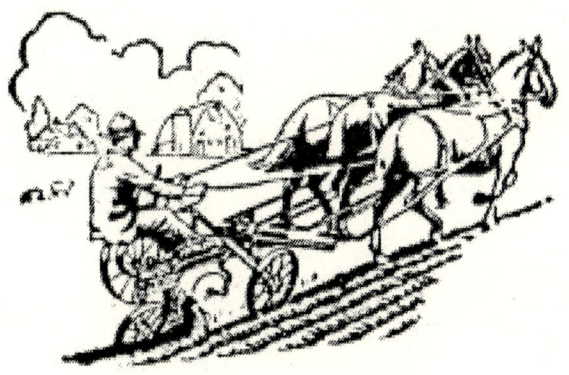

Life is a procession of problems that have to be addressed. Successful people address them as early as possible and as responsibly as possible.

Doc McDermith

Printed in the United States
928500002B